Praise for
Gina Meagher

"If you are living with a chronic medical condition, this book is for you. Although Gina lives with diabetes and celiac sprue, her insights and approach to life transcend her conditions. Everyone can benefit from her experience. Inspiring!"

~ KW, MD—Endocrinologist

"….. Gina takes you through the exploration of the journey to developing a personalized approach for managing diabetes. 'Know your body.' 'Advocate for yourself.' 'Don't let it define you.' These are among the concepts discussed as she reinforces discipline, perseverance, and triumph over difficult circumstances. As a medical professional, I gained more perspective and insight into the intricate journey of discovering, of managing, and of living with a chronic condition."

~ Karen F. Guess, MSN, ANP, PMH-NP, Doctoral Candidate

"..... Gina takes us through her journey of living with two chronic conditions and demonstrates how she continues to live life to the fullest and not let anything stand in her way. As a healthcare provider, I was inspired by Gina's message and I would recommend this book to other healthcare providers as well as to anyone living with a chronic disease."

~ Dr. Amy McIntosh, PT, DPT

"Wow, a super story, such good information... and easy to read. Thank you for sharing this with others! It is very encouraging! Bravo!"

~ Barbara Munson, Munson Communications

"I have long admired Gina for her can do attitude and her 'know thy self' spirit! Gina faces challenges head on and shares her learning with grace, courage and humility."

~ Susan McCarthy, Founder, Saol Development

The Nitty-Gritty of Managing Diabetes

The Nitty-Gritty of Managing *Diabetes*

Personalizing Your Approach
through Determination, Perseverance & Balance

Gina Meagher

The Nitty-Gritty of Managing Diabetes
Personalizing Your Approach through Determination,
Perseverance & Balance

Published by Something About Gina, LLC
info@somethingaboutgina.com

Copyright © 2017 by Gina Meagher
All rights reserved. No part of this book may be reproduced or transmitted in any form or by any means, electronic, mechanical, photocopying, recording, or otherwise, without prior written permission from Gina Meagher.

Book design by Kerrie Lian under contract with
Karen Saunders & Associates: www.KarenSaundersAssoc.com

Cover photo: iStock by Getty Images; Al Simonov

Printed in the United States of America
First Printing: November 2017

ISBN: 978-0-9886068-2-1 (paperback)
eISBN: 978-0-9886068-3-8 (e-book)

Library of Congress Control Number: 2017913309

The information in this book is not intended or implied to be a substitute for professional medical advice, diagnosis, or treatment. All content is for general information purposes only. The author makes no representation and assumes no responsibility for the accuracy of information contained herein. NEVER DISREGARD PROFESSIONAL MEDICAL ADVICE OR DELAY SEEKING MEDICAL TREATMENT. The author does not recommend, endorse, or make any representation about the efficacy, appropriateness, or suitability of any specific tests, products, procedures, treatments, services, opinions, healthcare providers or other information herein and THE AUTHOR IS NOT RESPONSIBLE NOR LIABLE FOR ANY ADVICE, COURSE OF TREATMENT, DIAGNOSIS, OR ANY OTHER INFORMATION, SERVICES, OR PRODUCTS MENTIONED HEREIN.

Stories shared are recalled to the best of the author's knowledge.

*To my husband, Jim,
who's always there for me.*

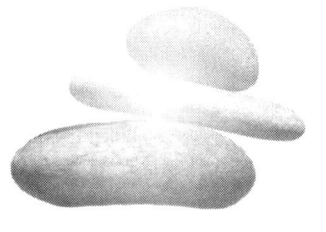

Table of Contents

Introduction i

Chapter 1: Something has Changed 1
  Own Your Own Power

Chapter 2: Beware of the Rabbit Hole 11
  The Importance of Attitude

Chapter 3: Know Thyself 19
  Your Management Has More to Do with You than Your Condition

Chapter 4: Levers and Pulleys 25
  One Size Doesn't Fit All

Chapter 5: Tools to Make Your Life Easier 33
  Management Options You'll Want to Consider

Chapter 6: The Dark Side 41
  The When and Where of Shot-Taking

Chapter 7: Dining Well 49
  Eat, Drink, & Enjoy Life

Chapter 8: Adventures Await You 61
  Being Confident Away from Home

Chapter 9: Leftovers 65
  Miscellaneous Topics I'm Frequently Asked About

Chapter 10: Letting Nothing Get in Your Way 83

Epilogue 87

Introduction

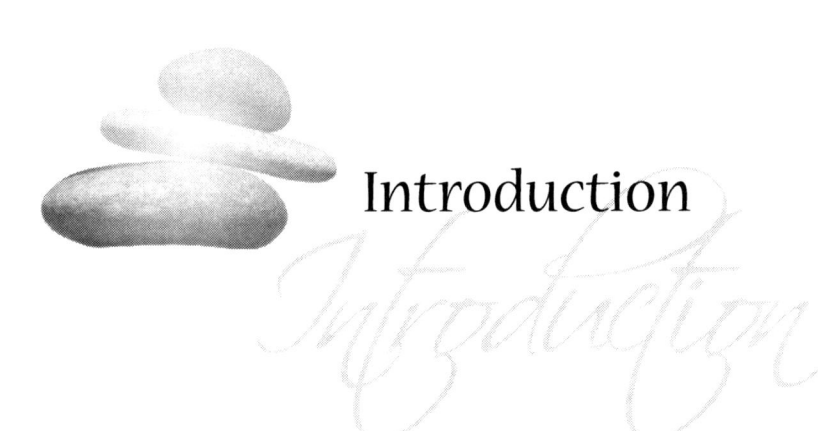

Ever since the release of my first book, *There Is Something about Gina: Flourishing with Diabetes and Celiac Disease*, people have been hinting to me about the idea of writing a second book. When I'd ask what, specifically, they'd want to read more about, it was always the same answer: more details about day to day management. The "nitty-gritty" of how to handle chronic conditions like celiac disease or diabetes, both of which I live with.

For the longest time, I hesitated. After all, a lot of the management process is very much dependent on what works on an individual basis. Yes, there are a few absolutes (if you're living with celiac disease, you need to avoid gluten, for instance, or if you're living with type 1 diabetes, you must take insulin and test your blood sugar), but so much is subject to individual preference that it seemed to me as if it would be next to impossible to write a book that would be right for any given personal approach. But then I realized that *that's* what management truly is (or should be) - a personal approach. And it occurred to me that a book about how to *personalize* one's approach to fit his or her particular circumstances or lifestyle could be a valuable book indeed.

In this book, you'll find many ideas that I trust you'll find useful, even valuable. As the title implies, this book covers the specifics of everyday chronic-disease management. Where my first book covered the forest (a more all-around view of living with diabetes and/or celiac disease), this one covers the trees. The nitty-gritty. But it does so keeping in mind that what works for me might not work for you. This book is more about options than rules. And I think you'll be surprised at just how many options there are. The key is to find the options that are right for you – for your condition, your personality, your lifestyle. In other words, this book is really about you and for you!

So, let's get started. Let's roll up our sleeves and get down to the nitty-gritty of managing *your* chronic condition.

1 Something has Changed

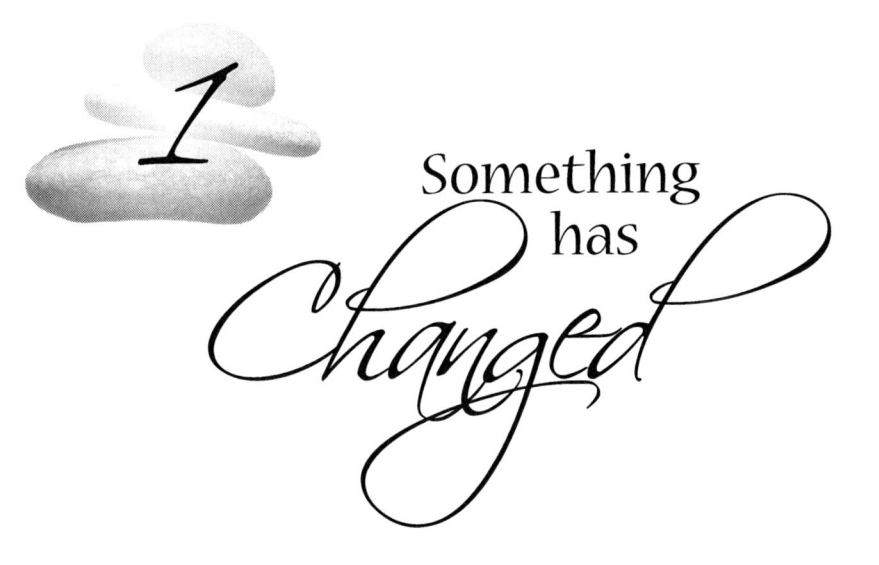

Own Your Own Power

In the course of writing this book, a book about the personalized management of chronic conditions, an incident happened that would have a significant impact on me and the management of my diabetes. If I had been looking for an example of how important it is to manage one's chronic condition given one's individual set of circumstances, I don't think I could have picked a better one. That doesn't mean I was happy about the sudden change in the state of my physical health, but at least it provided some lessons that we can make use of – a case study, if you will, illustrating the overarching theme of the book you're about to read.

It all began with an abnormality. That's what they called it. On the surface, that didn't sound so bad. What's a little abnormality? But shortly thereafter, I would learn that the "abnormality" would require nothing less than open heart surgery.

For someone living with diabetes, major surgery presents its own set of challenges when it comes to managing one's condition. And you do the best you can to take into account all of the factors (which we'll be discussing) that influence your blood sugar level so that you can respond accordingly. But open-heart surgery was a new ballgame for me. The surgery and the recovery that followed would present to me a real test of my management skills. Major surgery is stressful on the body for even the healthiest person. I could only imagine what kind of impact it would have on me, a person living with diabetes.

It started with a routine visit to my endocrinologist. I happened to mention that lately I'd been feeling a bit winded after certain activities, along with minor pain on the right side of my chest. I play recreational basketball and keep myself in decent shape, so the fact that it had become just a little harder to catch my breath after physically exerting myself was a concern. And it wasn't just after a hard game of basketball. I was finding myself a little winded after some fairly easy weekend walks with my husband, Jim, and even after walking from my car to my office at work each morning. Granted, it's not the shortest walk; we call it the "Long Green Mile" even though it's probably only about a quarter mile from the parking lot to my office. Still, the walk never used to leave me short of breath.

And then, about a month or so before my appointment with my endocrinologist, there was a particularly eye-opening experience. I was at a convention with my manager and we were walking from the convention center to the hotel, and I could not keep up with her, prompting her to ask, "Gina, what is wrong with you?" She knew me well, knew that it was not at all like me to struggle with an ordinary brisk walk. "You better get checked out," she said as I continued to lag behind her.

I wondered initially if it was just a case of my blood sugar being possibly too high or too low. But whenever I would test, my blood sugar would be between 90-110. I mentioned the development to my endocrinologist. "Maybe I just need to work out more," I suggested. After all, I knew I wasn't getting any younger.

"No," she said. "Something has changed, Gina. You should get an EKG." I set up an appointment with my primary care physician, who performed the EKG on a Friday, didn't entirely like what she saw, and then set me up with an appointment for a stress test the following Tuesday.

A stress test, if you've never had the pleasure, is undertaken on a slightly inclined treadmill that is further inclined a little more every three minutes or so. The goal is to raise your heart rate to a certain target rate that enables the doctor to observe your condition. Mine was a nuclear stress test, which means I was injected with a chemical called a radiotracer. From this, a visual image could be formed that showed the flow of blood into and out of my heart before the stress test, and then again afterwards, after about twenty minutes of rest.

It was at this point that the word "abnormality" was first mentioned. A further test – a cardiac catheterization (also known as an angiogram) – was then scheduled for that Friday. This test, I was informed, involved a dye injected into a catheter that would travel through my heart and reveal the extent of the blockage or blockages, which could then possibly be corrected with a stent.

Up until then, my level of concern had been relatively low. All the testing and procedures had been seemingly treated as routine by the doctors. But with each test, now culminating in the cardiac catheterization, I was becoming more and more aware of just how serious the situation might be. What began as a little short-windedness was starting to turn into an apparently major heart issue of some description. I was going from concerned to anxious.

On Wednesday afternoon of that week, the nurse from the center where I was scheduled for the catheterization called with some preliminary instructions. "The cardiologist doesn't want you taking any insulin on Friday morning before your procedure," she said.

"No insulin?" I replied. "I have to be honest with you; I'm not at all comfortable with that." I suggested that maybe the cardiologist had me confused with someone living with type 2 diabetes who might be able to go without his or her blood sugar medication for a morning. For me, as a type 1, I knew if I didn't take my insulin, my blood sugar would definitely spike. There was no getting around it. The doctor, naturally, was concerned about the opposite scenario – having me crash, dropping below 100 and continuing to drop. The best the nurse would do was check with the doctor and make a note on my chart about my concerns.

That evening, I emailed my endocrinologist, who agreed with my assessment and placed a call to the cardiologist on my behalf the next day. Then the cardiologist called me to discuss the matter further. Now, I have a great deal of respect for the medical profession and for the experience of this doctor. But the situation was one of those where, in my mind, you have to know your body and trust your instincts. The doctor, as skilled as he might have been, didn't know *me* the way that I know me. He made assumptions based on the average patient living with diabetes that he sees. There's nothing wrong with that. His experience with other patients is extremely valuable. But when medical advice is inconsistent with what you know about yourself, then you ought to speak up. This, I have come to learn, is a vital key to the management of any chronic condition.

At any rate, we talked on the phone and the cardiologist soon came to realize that I had a fairly good handle on the way that my body reacts to stress and responds to insulin. The key in his mind was that my blood sugar not dip below 100. You certainly don't want to deal with low blood sugar during a surgical procedure and so being a little on the high side is okay. That made perfect sense to me. We agreed that I would take half my usual amount of long-acting insulin the night before and that I would test myself in the morning and make an informed decision at that point as to whether or not to take additional insulin. He seemed comfortable with the idea that I was capable of doing so.

In the morning, my blood sugar was 301. High. And not at all surprising. Aware of the cardiologist's concern about me crashing during the procedure, but knowing my self, I took five and a half units of long-lasting insulin and two units of short-acting. When I arrived at the hospital for the procedure, my blood sugar was at 269 – going the right direction, but still quite high. While I was being prepped, the nurse took a phone call from the cardiologist, who was on his way in. He told the nurse to let me take whatever insulin I was comfortable taking. "Wow," she told me. "He never gives a patient that much of a say. You must really know what you're doing. You should teach a class!" I just had to smile.

I took two more units of short-acting insulin and right at the start of the procedure, I tested again. This time I was sitting at 211. Acceptable for the moment. I took no more insulin and about an hour or so later, I was at 147. Right before I was discharged, I was at 127. My management, knowing what I know about my body, was just right.

It's a question of knowing your body and how it reacts to situations. And then taking responsibility for managing your condition *while* balancing your medical team's knowledge and expertise. It's a collaborative approach. The key is to make sure whatever decisions you make are made with as much informa-

The Nitty-Gritty of Managing Diabetes

tion as you can gather. Knowing yourself and how your body works is a huge part of that.

In any event, the procedure itself brought some disconcerting news: three partial blockages on three main arteries, two full blockages on two minor arteries. "The blockages are too many and too extensive for the use of stents," the cardiologist told me. I would need bypass surgery. "I'm sorry," the cardiologist added, with a tone of genuine sincerity. "I know this isn't what you wanted to hear." *No !@#$% kidding!* I wanted to say.

The origin of my problems? Heredity. Heart disease runs on both sides of my family. But it would be naive of me to think that my diabetes wasn't a contributing factor. Regardless, all the doctors involved agreed that there was really nothing I could have done to have prevented my heart condition. This was good to hear; I didn't have to waste time blaming myself for somehow mismanaging my health.

The really good part of the equation was my relative youth and health and fitness. In fact, after my catheterization procedure, waiting in recovery, the surgeon who would eventually perform the bypass came in to see me and did a double take, checking his notes twice to make certain he had the right patient. Nurses would do the same. "*You* need a bypass?" It was nice to hear. Apparently, I didn't fit the profile. On the other hand, it didn't change the fact that I was now scheduled for major heart surgery. And I went from anxious to terrified.

Fortunately, the bypass surgery went well. There was no damage to the heart and the procedure was a success. Recovering afterwards, my initial problem was one of nausea, probably from the anesthesia. But then no form of pain medication agreed with me. And yet I had to eat to gain back my strength even though nothing tasted good to me. Eventually, except for foods with gluten, all my dietary restrictions were lifted so that I could get something down. I managed a little sorbet.

Of course, the other challenge was managing my blood sugar. Even without eating anything, my blood sugar was still running around 250 to 280, most likely due to the stress the situation produced. There's a common misunderstanding among patients newly diagnosed with diabetes that if you're not eating, you don't need to take insulin. But you must. In this case, my blood sugar remained high throughout my stay in the hospital despite the efforts of my medical team and me to lower it.

After five days in the hospital, I was sent home where even the slightest activities – dressing, showering, eating – would wipe me out. Jim started calling me the Queen of Naps. But little by little, my strength returned. I found initially that I had energy but was lacking in stamina. Eventually, that came back, too. It took time, but according to everybody on my medical team, that was to be expected. It could take a full year before I'd be able to return to my pre-surgery routine. Eventually, after six weeks of recovery, I was back at work. Part-time at first, and then after a couple weeks, I was working fulltime again. And just a couple months after that, I was back on the basketball court.

What I learned during the whole lengthy process is that coronary artery disease (an umbrella term for heart-related disease) is ten times more prevalent among people living with type 1 diabetes than people in the general population. But the connection is little understood. It's believed that the underlying factor is hyperglycemia, obviously an ongoing risk factor for those living with diabetes, but the experts aren't quite sure. My taking care of myself, my management of my diabetes, and my keeping in shape, likely prevented me from having heart problems earlier.

What prevented a heart attack was mentioning to my endocrinologist my concerns about my shortness of breath. It wasn't normal for me. In fact, at the very same convention where I couldn't keep up with my manager when we were walking to the hotel, my company had a rock-climbing wall set up for convention participants. I climbed it, but it was surprisingly hard for me and when I came down, my legs felt like jelly. I didn't have the strength initially to stand. I didn't even *want* to stand. I sat, waiting to catch my breath, taken aback by the strange feeling of intense fatigue. And although I tried to put these symptoms down to not being in as good a shape as I could have been, or simply to age, the fact is, something was wrong.

And this, I believe, is the key to not just managing one's chronic condition, but to managing one's health, no matter what conditions are present. You have to be in *sync* with your body. You should know what feels normal and what doesn't feel normal. Maybe, because of my diabetes, I've gotten a lot of practice at this, but the idea of being in sync is crucial for anybody's health. Problems, cardiac or otherwise, don't initially just step up and loudly announce themselves. But if you ignore them, they *will* grab your attention. For me, for instance, I learned that, without the surgery, I was probably only two to four months away from a heart attack. My boss and I talked afterward about how fortunate I was that nothing serious happened to me during that rock-climbing event. There are clues and you have to be paying attention to what your body is trying to tell you before it's too late.

When you're in sync, when you know your body, then you can act as your own advocate. You can question a doctor or second-guess a recommendation. Remember, just as with the cardiologist who directed me not to take any insulin the morning of my cardiac catheterization, doctors operate based on a set of assumptions that may or may not fit your situation.

It's a form of profiling and we all do it. We make assumptions in our everyday lives based on the way someone is dressed, for example, or what kind of car they drive, or how much they weigh, not to mention assumptions made based on race or gender. The medical field is no different. And the assumptions are made an indirect part of the treatment. But as my first endocrinologist once told me long ago, *not everything that happens to you is a result of diabetes.*

For instance, after my surgery, I struggled with nausea. No matter what nausea medication I was given, nothing seemed to help. The doctors and nurses more or less shrugged, determining that, because I was living with diabetes, I must have been suffering from gastroparesis, a condition where your stomach doesn't empty in a normal, timely way. People living with diabetes have an increased risk for gastroparesis. I've never had it, but no amount of my telling the doctors and nurses that would convince them my condition was anything else. Finally, once the nausea medication was out of my system, a nurse offered me a Tums. That cleared everything up just fine. Or maybe the nausea had simply run its course. Either way, the gastroparesis assumption was incorrect.

In fact, the general assumption on the floor as to why I was in the hospital in the first place was based – wrongly – on my diabetes. A couple of days after my surgery, the doctor was in my room giving a recap to some resident physicians and nurses.

I overheard a nurse say, "Yes, she's a diabetic."

I perked up. "Living with diabetes," I gently corrected her. (As you'll see, I don't especially care for labels when it comes to the chronic conditions I live with.)

"Yes, thank you," she acknowledged. But once "diabetes" was mentioned, I could sense an undercurrent from the residents and nurses, pointing to an assumption they were all making that my bypass surgery was a direct result of my mismanagement of my condition.

But then the doctor began to fill the others in. "Gina plays competitive basketball and manages her diabetes very well." I had to smile; it was "old-lady" basketball, at least that's what I called it, but who was I to argue with the doctor? The larger point, however, as the doctor explained, was that I was not at all a likely candidate for coronary artery disease, notwithstanding my diabetes. My problems were largely inherited. After the explanation, I could actually feel the tone in the room change. I was not just "a diabetic" with coronary artery disease. The assumed profile was off target. I was a person with multiple factors in play, all of which were important to the assessment of my overall health and well-being. From that point on, I was looked at a little differently. A little more accurately. In fact, I began being referred to on the floor as "the basketball player." And my subsequent cardio rehab sessions were designed to get me back on the court.

Remember: nobody's going to be an advocate for you but you. And if for some reason you can't be an advocate for yourself – if you're in a medical condition where you can't speak for yourself – make sure beforehand that your family has a firm grip on who you are and what you would want for yourself so they can properly advocate for you. When it comes to medical care, it's your responsibility to make sure that your medical team understands everything they need to know about you. And it all starts with *you* knowing about you.

2
Beware of the *Rabbit Hole*

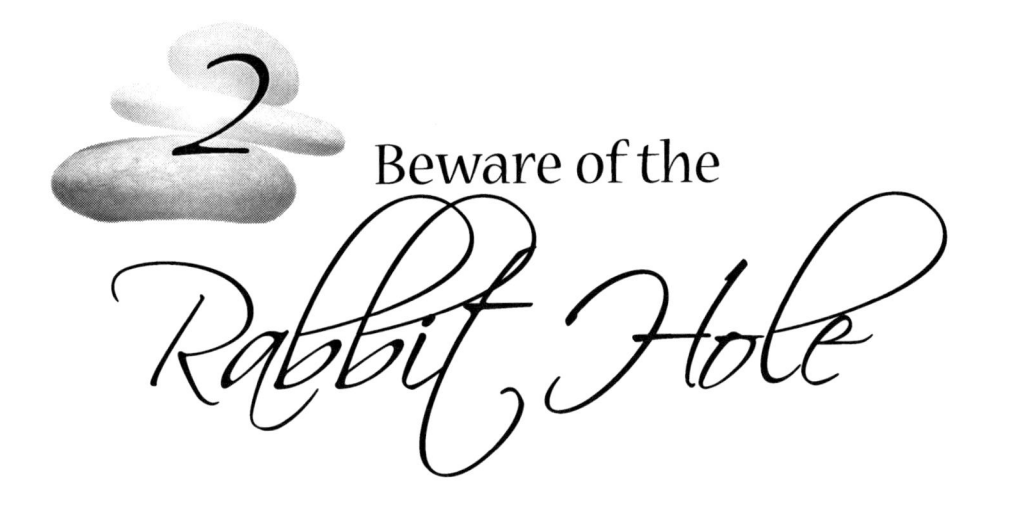

The Importance of Attitude

"Wow, Gina, you make it seem so easy!"

"Thanks," I always say. I know it's meant as a compliment. And the truth is that hearing it always brings a smile to my face. It makes me feel good about myself and about how I'm managing my chronic conditions – type 1 diabetes and celiac disease. But the fact is that it's not easy and at times I feel as if I want to explain to whomever paid me the compliment just how challenging it is to live with these conditions. Sometimes I feel as though my relative success is misleading and deceptive.

Still, I rarely find myself recounting the difficulties. Most people wouldn't want all the details, anyway. And a lot of people, not knowing exactly what to say, might feel helpless or uncomfortable. If only more people knew that just listening –

The Nitty-Gritty of Managing Diabetes

without judging and without saying *anything* – is a welcome response! And so, I mostly keep the specifics of my condition to myself. But there has been the rare occasion, with people who were genuinely interested and whom I trusted, when I took the time to share. For them, I felt a sense of wanting to let them know what's really involved.

One such occasion was when I shared my challenges with some friends I had become close to in a women's leadership group to which I belong. They all know I'm living with diabetes and celiac disease and one of them had off-handedly made the "you make it seem so easy" comment. But when I explained the truth, they were genuinely shocked at the efforts my management of the conditions requires. I described how a person living with diabetes has to always be thinking about where her blood sugar level is and was, what insulin she took and when, what she just ate, what she's going to eat, when she's going to eat it, what activities she's going to be engaged in, what activities she just finished, and all of the other factors that affect her glucose level.

"Sometimes," I confessed to them, "I just get tired of managing it. Really tired."

"Wow," they all said. "Gina, we had absolutely no idea."

I wasn't looking for sympathy. I was only trying to give them a perspective. But their compassion and support was touching, and it helped reaffirm for me the genuine kindness of most people.

I mention all this because if you're living with diabetes, celiac disease, or any chronic condition, I want you to know that I truly understand how difficult it is for you, both physically and emotionally. And although my intent with this book is to pass along some practical advice, I won't pretend that it's easy and I won't promise that I have all the answers, having somehow "mastered" the art of living with a chronic condition (or two).

This, too, is a frequent misunderstanding; one doesn't master a chronic condition any more than one controls it.

The problem with mastering a chronic condition is that the body is an incredible machine, complex and intricate and continually changing. Chronic conditions (or any health conditions, when you stop and think about it) are not simple and predictable. They do not come with quick and easy instructions. There are guidelines and strategies and most of the time they're generally effective. At times, they aren't. With diabetes, in particular, you're required to replicate the physical processes that other people's bodies perform naturally. And the body can often react in surprising ways, regardless of how careful or methodical you think you're being.

I prefer to think in terms of "managing" my chronic conditions, rather than controlling them. Managing is a more accurate term, and it's also more forgiving. Control is judgmental. There's a societal perception that plays a role. If my blood sugar is too high or too low, I am "out of control." I "cannot control" it. I'm not doing what I'm "supposed" to be doing. I'm not "compliant." Who needs that kind of pressure? In reality, nobody can manually control something as volatile and unpredictable as one's blood sugar with the same degree of sensitivity and accuracy as the body can on its own. So, you do the next best thing if your body is unable to do it. You do what you're capable of doing. You *manage* it.

Managing happens on two fronts: the physical considerations, of course, (which we'll delve more into later) but also the emotional ones. There is simply no way around the fact that living with a chronic condition can often be emotionally overwhelming. Sometimes it seems as though it's more than you can handle. It becomes exhausting. And you cannot control this feeling any more than you can control your disappointment when you don't get the promotion you were promised, the anger you feel when somebody cuts you off in traffic, or the fear you might feel walking down a dark street alone. These are normal emotions that are universal.

But we can *manage* these emotions. We can make sure our disappointment over the missed promotion isn't viewed as sour grapes and work on closing the gap in our experience, we can hold back our anger over the offending driver so that we don't react dangerously in traffic, and we can use our fear on the dark street to maybe pick up the pace a little and head for the safety of a more well-lit area. And we can certainly do our best to manage our emotions about a chronic condition as well.

Much of what we deal with on an emotional level comes from the perceptions of others. The vast majority of people will never understand what we go through every day. On the positive side, this might lead to observations about how "easy" we make it look. On the more negative side, we face insensitive or ignorant comments and behaviors.

My celiac disease, for instance, is misunderstood constantly. There is a difference between wanting to voluntarily cut back on gluten, and being gluten intolerant or having celiac disease where gluten presents an actual danger. Not everybody understands this. Once, at work, we were having a special luncheon. I always have a backup plan where food is concerned, making certain that I have something in my bag that I can eat if the food being offered isn't appropriate. In this case, I asked the person coordinating the luncheon if there was going to be a gluten-free option available so I could prepare properly. This annoyed her and I could tell from her reaction – a sigh and a roll of the eyes – that she thought I was being difficult. What's a little gluten, after all? ("Just take the croutons off the salad," is a good example of the kinds of comment I typically hear.) I even offered to call the caterer myself, thus relieving this woman of any inconvenience. That, too, was met with reluctance. She was the designated point-person and wasn't keen on delegating her responsibility. Protocol was protocol. After that, I just made myself a note to have something in my bag to eat that day.

Of course, I've had wonderful experiences, too. There was another colleague who had a similar attitude towards my celiac disease but who, over time, after learning more about my condition, became a strong advocate for me. She would make certain that my celiac disease would be taken into account during functions and company luncheons, or at least give me a heads-up, allowing me to prepare accordingly. She took the time to become educated, in other words, and over time her perception changed.

Living with diabetes brings on its own set of misperceptions. Because being overweight is one of the most well-known risk factors for type 2 diabetes, I'll sometimes hear, "You have diabetes? Funny, you don't *look* like you're a diabetic." I suppose this is meant as a compliment, but it just serves to reinforce to me how misunderstood my condition is. It's the same whenever I hear a comment about how all I have to do is "avoid sugar and take insulin." As if that's all it took. I wish!

These comments can bring an individual down. I'm sure you have your own stories. For me, the feeling of being left out is one of the hardest to emotionally deal with. Like, say, when everybody's in the break room eating cake for someone's birthday, but nobody bothered to ask Gina if she'd like a piece because the assumption is that her celiac and diabetes prevent her from eating any. It can be even worse if you're in a setting where not everyone knows you're living with a chronic condition. Bypassing me when offering cake to everybody else only serves to draw more attention to me. I become the focus of the room. Why isn't Gina being offered any cake? is suddenly the unspoken question. It's not that I want to hide my conditions. I am who I am. The point is that I don't want to feel excluded.

Offer me cake. Just like you would anyone else. It's nice to be asked; it's nice to be included. It's wonderful to be treated like everyone else.

If you're fortunate like me, these incidents are often balanced with moments of understanding and kindness. There are people at work who will make certain an option to the cake is available, for instance. These are the moments to focus on.

And we should be diligent about focusing on the positive. Being aware of all the negatives inherent in living with a chronic condition creates the potential for self-pity. It's okay to know what you're up against. But it doesn't do you any good to wallow and think of yourself as a victim. And yet it's all too easy to stumble into victimhood, to use your chronic condition as an excuse. But once you begin doing this on a regular basis, it becomes a habit that is difficult to break. And little by little, you'll cheat yourself out of whatever goals or dreams you might have, thinking that you're incapable of achieving them because you're a "victim" of a chronic disease that somehow makes you incapable of living to your fullest. This, not the condition, would be the real tragedy.

I certainly have days when I feel burdened and overwhelmed by the magnitude of my conditions. This I freely admit. But I never have days when I think I cannot do something I really want to do. I never have days when I think of myself as a victim. I never have days when I am ready to make excuses.

In fact, if you're like me, you find it especially infuriating whenever somebody makes an excuse *for* you based on your chronic condition. "Gina is a diabetic," I overheard a fellow colleague say to another. "She must be having a problem with her blood sugar today. That's why she was really short with you." I can understand a well-meaning defense of my actions, even if I don't need it. But sometimes, the defense isn't so well-meaning. Sometimes, as in this case, the excuse lacks genuine understanding. As it happened, on that particular day, I *wasn't* having a "blood sugar" problem. Instead, I had a full schedule and found myself up against a deadline on an important project. I was feeling a little stressed, like anyone might. I shared my frustration about the comment I overheard with a friend, who suggested I should have responded with, "So what's *your* excuse for acting like a jerk?" We laughed, but it was a good point. The fact is everybody has their moments. I won't ever use my conditions as an excuse, nor do I appreciate it when somebody else uses them that way, either.

This is not to suggest that my condition never impacts my day. Of course it does. There are times, although they're very rare, when my blood sugar level might be low (or high) and I just might not be feeling up to the task at hand. Every now and then, I might cut a meeting short, for instance, just like anyone might, and for their own personal reasons. "Do you mind if we pick this up a little later?" But, however my conditions impact me, I am fully responsible for the management of them and for taking care of myself. I take ownership for my actions.

And this carries over to my life outside of work as well. In the end, I am responsible for making certain I am enjoying life no matter what hurdles I come up against. It is this attitude that I am convinced allows me to not only survive with my conditions, but to flourish and thrive. And perhaps even more importantly, to maintain my positive outlook on life.

Do I stumble from time to time? Do I find myself teetering at the edge of the rabbit hole, ready to fall into the grip of burnout? Of course. We all do. So, what can we do? For me, I have come to learn how to identify those times when I might be in for an emotionally tough day. There are triggers, things that set me off and send me downward. You probably have them, too. Comments and behaviors from people – the exasperated woman who didn't want to take the time to ask if a gluten-free

The Nitty-Gritty of Managing Diabetes

option was available, the person making an excuse for me, the being left out – these are the kinds of situations that I know can get to me if I'm not careful. I don't look for them, but I know them when I see them, and the recognition helps me to process them and move on.

Recognize as well that if you're having one of "those" days, it's *one* of those days. Just one. Tomorrow will be brighter. Your immediate task at hand is simple: just get through the day. Try breaking the day down into smaller pieces. Get through the morning. Then get through the afternoon.

I have a mantra that I remind myself of: *Decide that just for today, nothing's going to stop you.* I start each day with this. Find one that works for you. Most days, I don't need it. Other days, I use it all the time, at least until it starts to take hold. Either way, it's always there if I need it. I'm almost always able to turn my day around. It might take an hour, maybe several, maybe most of the day. But sooner or later, I'm back on track, feeling strong and confident again.

Refuse to be a victim and refuse to make excuses for not enjoying life. Find the ways that work for you. Anticipate the triggers that bring you down. Know that most people do not understand your condition and be okay with that. Be ready for the comments. Refuse to be overwhelmed by the gravity of your chronic condition and, if need be, focus just on the day, or the morning, or the hour. Beware of the rabbit hole. Life is meant to be enjoyed, experienced, and shared. And remember that there aren't any excuses large enough to keep you from doing so.

3 Know Thyself

Your Management Has More to Do with You than Your Condition

When it comes to the management of a chronic condition, or conditions, it's important to bear in mind that much of the management comes down to a word you'll see used throughout this book: *personalization*. Your ways of managing will likely be completely different from someone else's, and yet both ways can be successful. As we continue to discuss effective management, remember that above all else, your style of management should be completely compatible with your personality. Proceed in a way that's consistent with who you are!

It's worth reflecting, then, on the respective strengths of different personalities. Knowing something about what kind of personality you have will help you manage your chronic condition(s) in ways that are right *for you*. And our distinctive personalities are marked by our different ways of thinking

The Nitty-Gritty of Managing Diabetes

and behaving. Dr. Geil Browning and Dr. Wendell Williamson of Emergenetics International (www.emergenetics.com) have identified four different preferences for how people think and three for how they behave. For our purposes here, in considering the best ways for an individual to personally manage his or her chronic condition, I would like to focus on the four "thinking" preferences. See if you recognize yourself in one (or more) of these preferences.

HOW I THINK: PERCENTAGES

ANALYTICAL = 25%
- Clear thinker
- Logical problem solver
- Data driven
- Rational
- Learns by mental analysis

CONCEPTUAL = 41%
- Imaginative
- Intuitive about ideas
- Visionary
- Enjoys the unusual
- Learns by experimenting

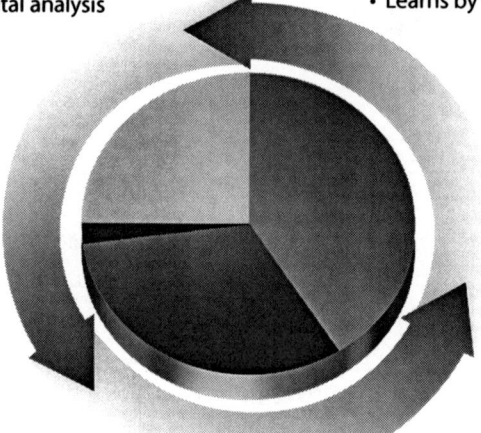

STRUCTURAL = 2%
- Practical thinker
- Likes guidelines
- Cautious of new ideas
- Predictable
- Learns by doing

SOCIAL = 32%
- Relational
- Intuitive about people
- Socially aware
- Empathetic
- Learns from others

The first is **analytical**. If you have an analytical preference, you're going to want to research your condition. You'll want to be informed and will therefore focus on gathering all of the data available to help you analyze and manage your condition. People with a **structural** thinking preference will prefer to have a practical, predictable, well-thought-out plan of action that they can manage and follow. Those with a **social** thinking preference will connect with their emotions and will likely manage their condition by engaging with others – family members or support groups. People with a **conceptual** thinking preference (me!) like to step back and see the whole picture and may find creative or unusual ways to manage their condition.

Most people have two or more of these preferences. I'm a conceptual thinker, but I also have social and analytical preferences. I can get a lot out of a conversation with my endocrinologist, for instance, because she is an analytical thinker. We talk about, for example, my blood sugar levels and trends and the effects on me of short- and long-acting insulin. We strategize, in other words, based on the data. We *analyze*, and that approach fits me well. On the other hand, I chafe against lists of do's and don'ts – what I can and cannot eat, for example. Lists, in and of themselves, aren't very helpful to me. Structural thinking would not at all describe how I think. I prefer to have the lists put into a context that makes overall sense to me. But because of my analytical preference, I also appreciate that the lists provide valuable information. In other words, know the strengths of your personality type, but guard against the challenges, too.

The point is to be aware of how you best process information. If you're a structural thinker you might like and benefit from the lists that I chafe against and you might feel more comfortable adhering to the plan and following the rules to the letter. And that's perfectly okay. If you're analytical, you might decide to do a lot more research and find other ways to manage your condition in addition to those detailed here. Go for it. If you're a social thinker, you might prefer learning from the experiences of others whom you've read about or met in person. Find the ways to manage your condition that enable you to work through your strengths and allow you to optimize the gift of your unique personality. In other words, be yourself. Don't try to be somebody you're not. Managing is hard enough without having to reinvent yourself.

Personalization, of course, doesn't mean doing whatever you feel like doing. When I was first diagnosed with diabetes, I was bombarded with information about what I should and should not eat. These were the lists of do's and don'ts that I initially resisted. Over time, however, I came to realize that if I was going to live my life the way I wanted, I needed to make a few concessions. Some allowances. That's just the way it is. I had to be realistic. You should know and respect your body's limitations with respect to your chronic condition. You *have* to do your best to make lifestyle changes and there is simply no getting around this fact.

Once I understood this, I accepted it. When it came to my dietary restrictions, for instance, making changes wasn't all that intolerable. After all, eating whatever I want to eat, however much I want, and whenever I want to eat it aren't high priorities for me in the grand scheme of things. What's important to me is experiencing and enjoying life to the fullest. If my blood sugar is always high, or if it's always low, I'm going to feel miserable – tired and lethargic. That's going to directly affect the quality of my life. Forgoing foods that wreak havoc with my glucose levels is a small price to pay for the ability to live the life I want to live.

I came to think of it like this: there are certain foods I *choose* not to eat. I never think I *can't* eat them. That's much too negative and limiting. And if you're like most people, if somebody says you can't do something, your initial reaction is to want to do it, even if you'd never even thought of doing it before! It's human nature. So, I give myself permission to eat anything I want; I simply choose not to eat certain things. My focus, in fact, doesn't even go towards foods I choose not to eat. For both my celiac disease and diabetes, my focus stays entirely on the foods that I *can* eat.

If I get a craving for a specific food that I just can't ignore, I might allow myself a small taste of it. I know, for example, that sometimes I get an urge for a Dairy Queen Peanut Buster Parfait. A temptation I simply cannot resist. But I can pretty easily talk Jim into ordering one and then letting me have a spoonful or two of it. Maybe even three. This satisfies my craving. It's the feeling of being deprived, the idea of never being able to eat *any* of a certain food, that can get depressing. A spoonful or two (or three) of a Peanut Buster Parfait reminds me that I am still in charge, in that I at least still have the freedom to decide. The freedom to choose is empowering. I will always choose wisely (I won't eat a whole Peanut Buster Parfait, and even with just a couple of spoonfuls, I might take an extra unit of insulin – or two – to accommodate) but the decision will be mine, and this makes all the difference. And, ironically, I have found over time that once I give myself permission to eat a certain food, I don't seem to want it as much. It's the blanket prohibition of it that often makes it more desirable!

What I've come to realize over time is that the guidelines for what to eat and what not to eat and how much are only that – guidelines. Nothing is written in stone. The reason for this is simple: everybody is different. What might have a huge effect on one person might have little or no impact on another. The guidelines are a very good start – a valuable foundation. But they're just a start. Knowing yourself, and knowing how your body reacts, are keys to the appropriate management of your condition. For that allows you to make the necessary adjustments. And it also allows you to color outside the lines from time to time, to cross the boundaries of the guidelines, at least a little.

For example, in our house, Saturdays are not just Saturdays. Jim has declared them "Pancake Saturdays." If we're not busy with other weekend plans or traveling somewhere, Saturday starts off with a pancake breakfast. Knowing how a pancake breakfast affects me helps me to properly prepare for it. I might take an extra unit or two of short-acting insulin. I'll also try to anticipate what other activities I'll be engaged in that day. Are Jim and I planning a hike later? A bike ride? A movie? Are we planning on just relaxing?

When you learn to properly personalize your approach, you won't be stuck governing your life to accommodate your chronic condition. You'll be successfully managing your chronic condition to accommodate your life. For me, I will not allow my diabetes to affect what's really important to me – the priorities in my life. What I *will* do is make the necessary allowances. By doing so, I can lead the full – and healthy – life I wish to lead.

4
Levers and Pulleys

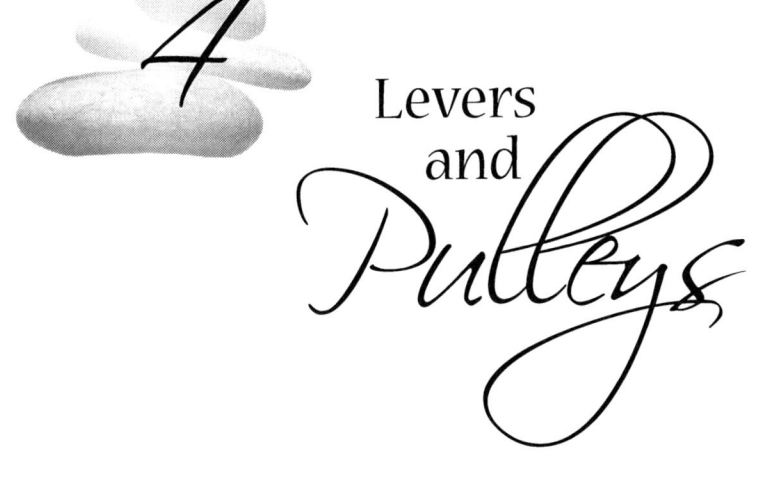

One Size Doesn't Fit All

For the management of my diabetes, the general objective is to keep my blood sugar as close as possible to where it would be for a person not living with diabetes, which is 80 to 120. But I give myself some leeway. Somewhere between 90 and 140 is okay with me. I'd rather be a bit high than low, guarding against the chance of going even lower, which can result in a rebound effect. (We'll discuss rebounding later.) That's not to say if I'm at 140, I won't try to get my blood sugar lower. Of course I will. But I'm not going to panic at 140, or beat myself up over it. In other words, I give myself permission to fail. You learn to be flexible and know where your comfort level is. More than anything, you should get yourself to the point where you're okay with the idea that you might not always be perfect. That's just the nature of the condition. Remember: you're trying to figure

The Nitty-Gritty of Managing Diabetes

out intellectually what the pancreas of a person without diabetes does automatically. It's not going to be easy.

Having said all that, it's not impossible and there are many steps you can take to empower yourself. Again, it starts with knowing your body and how it reacts. And this takes experience. A lot of trial and error. There are several crucial factors that can help, including knowing your carbohydrate ratio, your correction factor (insulin sensitivity factor), your reaction time to insulin, and your level of physical activity. These are key. You simply have to know them for the successful management of your condition. And all of these factors need to be balanced and taken into account. Everything has to work together. Although they're separate factors, they're constantly interacting and should be given equal weight. It's a series of levers and pulleys, each having an effect on the other and each having an overall effect on your blood sugar.

Your **carbohydrate ratio** is how much insulin your body requires to cover a given amount of carbs. A very general rule of thumb (and useful if you're just starting out) is that 1 unit of short-acting insulin will cover 15 grams of carbs (one carb exchange). Over time, you'll determine a more accurate and personalized number by analyzing your glucose readings before and after meals. I eventually learned that my carb ratio is closer to 1 to 10. So, if I know a meal I'm about to eat is going to consist of 30 grams of carbs, that – for me – means 3 units of insulin. I also know that late in the day, around dinner, my carb ratio is 1 to 8. It varies, in other words, during the course of the day. In the evening, I'm more likely to be less active. And so, I take more insulin at dinner than at lunch or breakfast, for the same amount of carbs. Of course, you must know the amount of carbs. You have to become diligent about reading food labels. I've become an expert, but naturally I didn't learn any of this overnight. I paid attention and now I have a pretty solid idea of my carb ratio which helps me to more accurately gauge what my insulin requirements are to keep my blood sugar between 90 and 140.

An especially useful guideline to correct for high blood sugar (which you *will* experience), based on your total daily insulin dose or your TDI, is what's called the Rule of 1800. This **correction factor** tells you how many mg/dl your blood sugar will drop (approximately) for 1 unit of short-acting insulin, given your TDI. The formula looks like this:

1800 ÷ TDI = mg/dl drop per short-acting insulin unit

For example, suppose my total daily insulin dose (both short- and long-acting) is 40 units. 1800 ÷ 40 = 45. This means I can expect my blood sugar will drop by 45 with a single unit of insulin. Obviously, this is handy to know. But like any guideline, your results will likely be different. The important message here is to learn how this guideline works for you. Maybe, on average, your drop is closer to 40. Or 50. In time, you'll know.

I've also come to understand what I refer to as my body's **reaction time** (the time it takes for the insulin to start working) with respect to taking insulin and with respect to eating. There are useful guidelines available based on the type of insulin you take (e.g., duration, peak, etc.). But, always looking to personalize my management, I have, over time, been able to construct a table that helps me coordinate both my eating and taking insulin. If my blood sugar is high, I want to give the insulin a chance to start working (a head start, if you will) before I eat. Conversely, if my blood sugar is low, I'll want to eat sooner rather than later. Adjusting the timing of my eating relative to the timing of my shot gives me a big edge in managing my blood sugar level.

The Nitty-Gritty of Managing Diabetes

Blood Sugar Level	Timing of Shot	Timing of Eating	Correction Factor
≤80 (mg/dl)	After Eating	Right Away	N/A
81-150	Before Eating	Within 10 Mins. of Shot	0-1
151-200	Before Eating	Wait 10-15 Mins.	1-2
201-250	Before Eating	Wait 15-20 Mins.	2-3
>250	Before Eating	Wait 30 Mins.	≥3

What the table does is allow me to gauge how many units of short-acting insulin I may need in addition to what I normally take. If, for example, I roll out of bed and see that my blood sugar is under 80, I know I need to eat breakfast right away. I'll delay giving myself my first shot of short-acting insulin until after I eat. If, let's say, before lunch my blood sugar level is up around 160, then I know I need to take my shot right away. And I'll probably need a single unit of extra insulin to correct for the higher-than-desired level. Closer to 200, and I might take two extra units. I've also learned that, for me, to give the insulin time to work, I will put off lunch somewhere between 10 and 15 minutes (still assuming a level of 160). Up around a 250 level, I'll need closer to three extra units and I'll wait closer to 20 minutes before I eat.

These numbers might not work at all for someone else, but they work well for me. I learned them through experience. And in fact, I learned them so well that this table was just floating around in my head for years before I ever bothered to reduce it to writing. When you consistently take your blood sugar readings and pay attention, you can construct your own table. Like me, you may not need to write it out, either. After a certain amount of time and experience, you'll just know.

I always bear in mind, however, that the numbers in the table, appropriate for me at this point in my life, can (and will) change. They've held relatively steady for awhile now, but over the long haul of your life, your body changes, your medical condition changes, you go through periods of more or less stress, your level of physical activity changes, and other factors pop up that can have an effect. All of this means that your reaction time to food may change as well. Just a reminder to always be open to reviewing and reevaluating your strategies.

Knowing your carb ratio, knowing your correction factor, and knowing your reaction time are all important ways to properly adjust your insulin intake for various situations. But there's another factor that can affect how your body reacts to insulin and that's your **activity level**. In general terms, physical activity, like exercise, will lower your blood sugar level. So, you might choose to eat a carbohydrate and a protein first. Or maybe have an energy drink or juice. Sometimes, I might even take less insulin to compensate for the activity. But adjusting for physical activity is highly personal, varying from one individual to the next. And even from one type of activity to the next for any given individual.

As with the other factors, you just need to pay attention and learn your own tendencies. With me, for example, I've discovered that if I play basketball, I can expect my blood sugar to initially rise and then drop a little bit within two to three hours. If I play a round of golf, on the other hand, I can expect my blood sugar to drop during the course of the round. So, I'll make adjustments accordingly. On the other hand, I've noticed that – with me – if my blood sugar is above 250, physical activity can actually make my blood sugar *rise*. So, in this case, I'll wait until my blood sugar has dropped to under 200 before I engage in exercise. Again, it's all a matter of personal tendencies.

In general, before I do anything that requires at least moderate physical activity, including walking, I target my blood sugar to be somewhere between 100 and 150. The goal, of course, is to not drop too low (less than 80). So, no matter what activity I plan on being engaged in, I'll make sure I have something with me to eat or drink if need be.

In the meantime, of course, any adjustments I make still need to consider the other factors – the carb ratio, for instance, or the typical reaction time, or the correction factor. In the example above where I find myself at 160 and decide to take an extra unit before lunch, I might just forego that extra unit if I'm planning a physical activity shortly thereafter.

By the way, while we're on the subject, you probably don't need me to tell you about the advantages of physical activity. It's important to understand, though, that you don't need to train like an athlete. You don't need to play basketball or run or hike long distances. Going for a walk or doing some gardening are examples of low-impact activities that nevertheless can make a difference. Daily exercise is ideal, but there's nothing wrong with engaging two or three times a week in some kind of physical activity. Find something you like and do it! Who knows? You might just start making it a daily habit.

When it comes to managing your condition, there are plenty of other factors to consider. Emotional stress, for example. Illness. Surgery. Over-the-counter medications. Even just fighting off a cold. If you're a woman, you might notice, like I have, that your blood sugar is impacted by your period. It can be impacted by pregnancy, too. And, on top of all of that is the effect that certain foods might have and/or the portion sizes of those foods. We'll talk later about management and the importance of taking into account specific foods. For now, it's important to understand that proper management means balancing a whole lot of factors that may be impacting your body at any given time. It's a continuous *process*, in other words. If it sounds a bit overwhelming, well, it is. But you can get through it. By paying close attention to how your body reacts – and with experience, trial and error, and patience – management becomes a lot less overwhelming.

And to start, regardless of the multitude of factors, remember the main ones: your carb ratio, your correction factor, your reaction time to insulin, and your level of physical activity and how physical activity affects you. In fact, over time, I've learned that I can even narrow it down further and say that my carb ratio and level of physical activity are the factors that have the biggest effect on me and my blood sugar levels. But it's important to understand the other factors, too. It's often a question of prioritizing. You'll learn what impacts your blood sugar the most and, over time, you won't feel quite so overwhelmed. Your management will become second nature.

Now, am I always perfect? Hardly! Sometimes, despite my best efforts, and despite how well I think I know myself, I have times when all of my efforts fall short for no explainable reason. It's frustrating, but it happens. But that's okay. An aberration here and there is not unusual. It becomes an issue only if what you're trying fails to work consistently. If you're routinely over 150, for example, or less than 80, no matter what you do, then you should take the time to understand why.

Are you experiencing these particular blood sugar readings only at certain times of the day? After certain foods? Certain activities? What's the trend? Or might some of the many other factors be in play? What's the common thread?

The Nitty-Gritty of Managing Diabetes

Figure out the trigger, and you can make the proper adjustment. And remember that your medical team can be a great resource in helping you to get a handle on what might be throwing you off. Once a trigger or pattern is uncovered, you'll have one more piece of information that can help you in the future. After awhile, you'll have a mental list of all your triggers and it will be that much easier next time to get yourself back on track.

Remember to be patient. Don't be discouraged if you don't know exactly how to make the proper corrections right away. It'll come. The challenges of management are not insurmountable. But proficiency doesn't happen overnight either. It took me years and I'm still learning. And just when I think I've got it nailed, I'll often find that I need to do some recalibrating. And frequently, often right back to where I was before! It's an ongoing process. Just like life itself, it's a journey.

Another thing to remember is to not panic. It's easy to over- or under-correct, taking too much or too little insulin. This puts you on a roller-coaster. Better to make small adjustments and observe what happens than to make big adjustments that swing you too wildly in the other direction, requiring yet another adjustment. Do your best to resist changing more than one factor at a time. If you do, you won't really know which correction was responsible for the result of the change.

And when you make an adjustment, wait two or three days to gauge the true results. You're managing for the long term, after all. We're talking about a lifestyle. Being patient and learning how a particular adjustment affects you gives you another piece of valuable information you can add to your tool belt. The process *will* get easier with time and practice. Trust me. Today, my management has just become second nature. It certainly doesn't define me; it becomes a part of who I am and what I do.

5
Tools to Make Your Life *Easier*

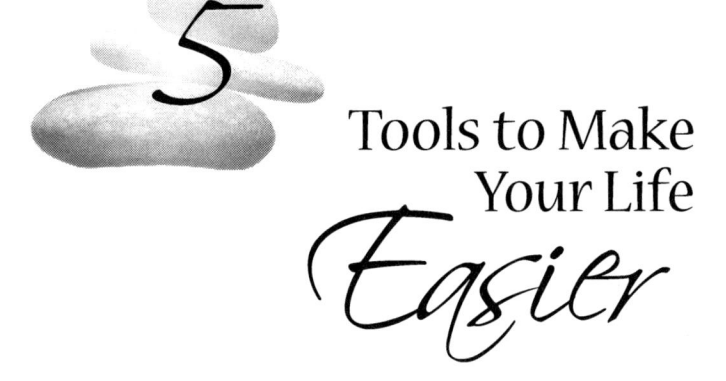

Management Options You'll Want to Consider

There's an old Frank and Ernest cartoon by Bob Thaves about Fred Astaire where someone says, "Sure, he was great, but don't forget that Ginger Rogers did everything *he* did...backwards and in high heels!" The proper management of a condition like diabetes reminds me of this cartoon. Going through life with diabetes is like dancing backwards in high heels. It's just that much more challenging. But of course, that doesn't mean you can't be a great dancer. And living with diabetes doesn't mean you can't live life to the fullest. It just takes a bit more effort than it might for the person who's not living with diabetes. And that effort comes down to proper management.

In the last chapter, we discussed learning how to make insulin adjustments based on your own body and how it reacts to various stimuli (carbs, physical activity, etc.). Just as important is the decision of how you want to go about administering your insulin. Once upon a time, there wasn't much personal choice in the matter. You used a single-use syringe and there was only one kind of insulin available. But times have changed and today, there are a few more options to consider, including the pump and the pen. I've used them all.

Whereas a syringe is used to inject long-acting insulin (basal) once or twice a day drawn up from a vial, followed by short-acting insulin injections at mealtimes (bolus) or when needed (there are some insulins that can be combined and injected at the same time), an insulin pump works by delivering short-acting insulin all day long through an infusion set inserted under your skin. Pumps are programmable, allowing you to manage the amount of insulin for different times of the day and for meals, etc. You can program for additional insulin when needed (maybe to cover a few extra carbs in your dinner, or just when you have higher than expected glucose levels). Some people find that making it this convenient to correct their blood sugar level means they're more apt to do it. It's the pressing of buttons versus pulling out a vial and a syringe (or pulling out a pen and dialing in the dosage).

When they were new, as I well remember, pumps were much bigger and heavier than they are today, about the size of a paperback book compared with the size of a cell phone, and with flexible tubing that ran from the pump to the spot of insertion. Today, there is even a pump that can be worn right at the spot of insertion, on the abdomen, arm, or leg, for instance. (These types of pumps are controlled by a wireless remote device that you can carry around in your pocket or purse.) And so, whether it's a pump attached to your body, or one with flexible tubing, it's much easier to carry around a pump today. It's easier to conceal one, too. You can clip it onto your belt, hide it in a pocket, a waistband, a bra, even thigh-highs.

I've always liked the pump but I've never personally cared for the idea of having something tethered to my body twenty-four hours a day, seven days a week. Still, I had gotten used to wearing a pump long ago when they first came out. My particular brand, unfortunately, was recalled due to a manufacturer's defect and I just never went back to the pump. It was hard initially to return to the idea of shots but now that I've been back on shots so long, I've been reluctant to go back to the pump. But I'm currently revisiting the idea based on what we'll discuss in a bit.

Insulin pens combine the syringe and insulin into a single delivery device that's even more portable and less obvious than pumps. These devices look like large marking pens. Reusable pens come with disposable cartridges that contain up to 300 units of insulin. There are disposable ones, too, that carry the same amount, but you throw the pen out when the insulin is gone. Normally you can buy a package of five at a time. I like the pen but it can be a bit pricey and it so happens my insurance doesn't cover it. Certainly, when you're trying to decide what is right for you, cost plays a role.

In any event, whether you use a syringe, a pump, or a pen, the bottom line is that these are just tools for your management. They won't manage your blood sugar for you. The management is up to you. A pump, for instance, can help you determine the amount of insulin to take based on your carb ratio, correction factor, etc., but you still have to provide those inputs. You still have to be in tune with your body and you still have to take all the factors into account that we discussed earlier. There are no shortcuts.

Just as there are options for the delivery of insulin, there are options for something just as important: the monitoring of your blood sugar. After all, you can't make an informed decision about your treatment plan without knowing where you're starting from or where you've been or where you're trending.

There are several types of *glucometers* on the market, each designed to allow you to get a reading on your blood sugar. They come with distinctive features and you'll need to find the one that's right for you. What are the features you find most important? Cost might be a factor for you. Most glucometers are fairly inexpensive, but you might want to consider the price of the test strips that are used with any given glucometer. Prices on those can vary widely. Data source capability might also be important to you; with some monitors, you can download the readings to a computer or smart phone. You can have your doctor download them as well. Some monitors have audio if you're visually impaired. Button sizes differ. So do screen sizes. Find what you're most comfortable with.

Then there are the *continuous* glucose monitors (CGMs). These also measure your glucose level but are wearable like the insulin pumps. Typically, they can be worn for up to seven days at a time with a disposable sensor that's inserted under your skin. There's a transmitter that connects to the sensor that sends the glucose readings wirelessly to a receiver, mobile phone, or an insulin pump. But a CGM has to be used in conjunction with your glucometer, which is used to calibrate it.

The calibration is necessary because CGMs aren't quite as accurate as good old-fashioned finger-stick glucose monitoring. In fact, the FDA has yet to approve the CGMs as an acceptable substitute, although manufacturers are working with the FDA on this. Soon, no doubt, the technology will be such that the need for finger-stick testing will be reduced and ultimately eliminated. CGMs measure glucose levels in the tissue, whereas a glucometer measures glucose levels in the blood. But once calibrated to an accurate finger-stick reading using your glucometer, they work fairly well, typically plus or minus 30 points. While you're wearing a CGM, it will measure your glucose level every five minutes. In this way, you can more accurately and more easily spot trends, which is much more difficult to do if you're just measuring your glucose level with a glucometer at, say, meal times and at bedtime, as most people do.

As a result, you can make adjustments that you might not otherwise make. For example, it's frustrating when you haven't changed anything about your routine or food intake and yet for some reason you see your blood sugar level changing dramatically from one day to the next. Maybe you eat the same food every day for breakfast and suddenly, out of nowhere, your blood sugar readings are different at lunch than they were the day before. One day maybe your blood sugar is much higher than normal; one day maybe it's much lower.

For example, I often eat cottage cheese and fresh fruit and a piece of toast for breakfast. One day my blood sugar might be 100 in the morning and 100 at lunch. No problem. But then the next morning, same 100 reading in the morning, same breakfast, and a blood sugar reading of 50 at lunch! The morning after that, 350 at lunch! What's going on? The fewer readings you take, the more difficult it is to anticipate where your level is going to be. It's hard to make a prediction if your situation is suddenly unpredictable. A continuous glucose monitor allows you to track what's happening to you *as it's happening*. And then you can accommodate appropriately, and in a timely way. This, of course, is a huge advantage. With a CGM, I won't be surprised by a 50 or 350 reading at lunch because I'll be observing the fall or rise in real time. Most importantly, I'll know to do something about it beforehand, thus helping me to level out the frustrating ups and downs.

Some people wear a continuous glucose monitor twenty-four hours a day, seven days a week. My preference is to wear one for a week at a time and then give myself a break for a week. Wearing it for a week helps me to get a handle on what's happening with me. Then I'll apply what I've learned, making the proper insulin and food adjustments. When I take a week off from the CGM, I'll still measure my glucose regularly with the glucometer.

Keep in mind that you can roughly mimic the results of a CGM with a glucometer simply by taking frequent readings, like once an hour. But just as the convenience of the insulin pump means you're more apt to correct your glucose level than if you have to take the time to pull out a vial and syringe or a pen, the convenience of the CGM means you're more apt to keep track of your glucose level than if you have to repeatedly check it with a finger stick test. But it's all a matter of personal preference. If you're like me and you don't like the idea of having something attached to your body all day long, you might decide the CGM is not for you. Or, like me, you might decide to just wear one for a few days at a time.

Some CGMs today can interface with insulin pumps. With some of them you can program the pump to, for example, automatically suspend insulin for a certain amount of time if the CGM determines that your glucose level has dropped to a certain level. This is a real game-changer. A CGM interfacing with a programmable pump is the closest you can get to doing what your pancreas and brain are supposed to do automatically. But, again, this will only work for you if you're comfortable with the idea of having something attached to your body all the time. That doesn't exactly describe me, as I mentioned earlier. But here is where I'm doing a bit of rethinking. The relatively recent technology that allows for the interfacing of pump and CGM might just be worth the trade-off.

Even with all the innovative technologies (including new apps that are seemingly being created every day), I want to reiterate that there is no substitute for your own hands-on management. If you're thinking that a pump, interfacing with a CGM, is a substitute for management, bordering even on a cure, then you're probably not a suitable candidate for it. In fact, many people find their management becomes even more involved with a CGM and pump because they're able to see the information they need in real time, thus empowering and enabling them to respond more quickly to changes in glucose levels. The up-to-the-minute information means they have more flexibility. But of course, that entails more hands-on management. The tools are there to help you manage; they're not there to take over the management for you.

Whether it's a tool to help with the delivery of insulin or a tool to help you monitor your glucose level, find what works *for you*. Use the tools that you feel comfortable using. Shop around and compare. And remember that advances are being made all the time. In today's Internet age, it's easy enough to keep yourself up to date with everything that's available to help you manage your diabetes. Monitors, pumps, pens, syringes, infusion sets, even lancing devices – they come in many different styles with many different features. Way too many to cover here. The main idea is to determine which features are important to you and do your homework. Visit the manufacturers' websites. Read online reviews from other users. Talk to people in your support group, family, or friends who might also be living with diabetes. Also, check out *Diabetes Forecast*, the bimonthly magazine from the American Diabetes Association. And don't forget to consult your own medical team – always a great resource.

6

The Dark Side

The When and Where of Shot-Taking

It's funny what people think about needles. Universally, nobody likes them. With some people, it's more of a phobia. Whether it's a tetanus shot or a flu vaccine or a blood test, the sight of that needle seems to make people cringe. I was reminded of this at a dinner event. I was seated at a table with Jim and several other people, some of whom I didn't know. I don't remember how the subject came up but one of the people began to talk about her friend who was living with type 2 diabetes. The friend was apparently trying to manage her condition with exercise, by paying close attention to what she ate, and by taking oral medication – trying to do whatever she could to avoid having to take insulin injections.

"I mean, who wants to take shots all the time?" this person at the table said. "Can you imagine how horrible that would

The Nitty-Gritty of Managing Diabetes

be?" And I knew there was more going on with her friend's reluctance – and her understanding of her friend's reluctance – than just the unpleasant use of a needle.

There's a perception with people living with type 2 diabetes that if you resort to taking insulin injections, instead of oral medication or making changes to your diet or exercising, you're somehow failing at keeping your diabetes in check. Your diabetes is getting the better of you and you're mismanaging it. The same idea exists with type 1 diabetes (in which case you *must* take insulin injections) where the perception is that the larger the dose of daily insulin you need, the worse you are at managing your condition. But these are *huge* misperceptions. Diabetes is much more complex than that. Whether you're living with type 1 or type 2, you manage your diabetes any way you need to and by any means necessary. And you manage in a way that works for you, not anybody else. Whatever you have to do – diet, exercise, oral meds, x or y units of insulin a day – all that matters are the results. You cannot, and should not, manage by the standards or perceptions of others. Manage for what is right for you.

Now, of course this woman at the table didn't know I was living with diabetes and I noticed Jim and some of the others sort of glancing over at me as the story was being told, probably wondering what I was thinking. I thought I'd better lighten the moment so I said, jokingly, "Yeah, who wants to go over to the dark side?"

"Yes!" she exclaimed. "That's it! The dark side!" Everybody laughed and soon enough the conversation moved on to other topics.

There was a time, after I'd just been diagnosed, when taking shots was anything but a laughing matter. But now, years later, taking shots is something I do almost without thinking. The moments of cringing or wincing just before I inject my insulin are long behind me.

This fact is always surprising to people because as difficult as it is for most people to take a shot (like a flu shot), it's even more difficult for them to imagine having to administer a shot to themselves. Or, unless the person is a nurse or doctor, to administer a shot to somebody else.

"What's it like to give a shot?" my niece asked me one time when she was just ten. She knew I'd been living with diabetes and she saw me one evening getting ready to inject myself.

"Well, Sarah," I said, "do you want to try it? You can give me a shot."

"Sure!" she said, very enthusiastically. Of course, I was a little apprehensive, wondering to myself if this was really a good idea, after all. Was Sarah going to push the needle nice and steadily into me, or was she going to stab me with it? Sarah's mother, a nurse by profession, was present and she must have felt the same because I could see her eyeing us anxiously. But I knew it was a good teaching moment and I wanted Sarah to experience the entire process, a little slice of my everyday routine.

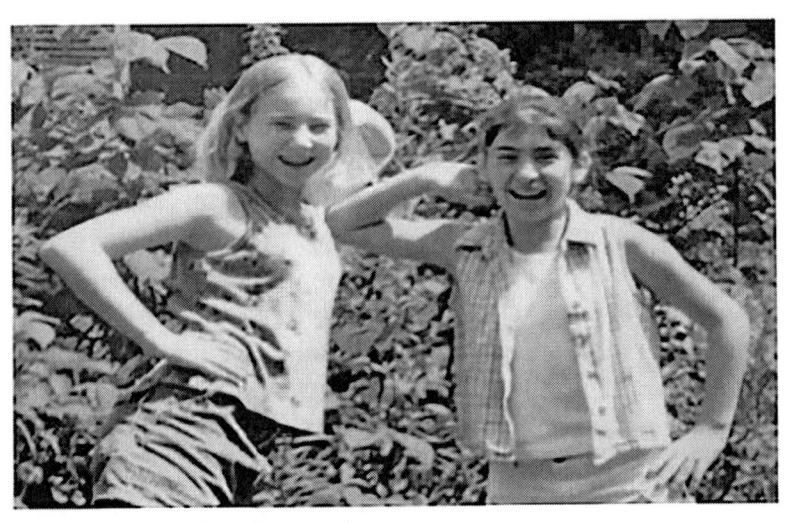

My nieces – Sarah and Amanda

The Nitty-Gritty of Managing Diabetes

I explained to Sarah that I had to take shots to compensate for the fact that my pancreas didn't naturally produce insulin like hers did. First, I had her test her own blood sugar, which of course was within an acceptable range (although I strangely found myself feeling a little uneasy, wondering what I'd do or say if it wasn't!). And then I had her test my blood sugar. Next, I had her measure the dose of insulin, told her how to draw the insulin from the vial, showed her how to tap the air bubbles out of the syringe, and then explained how to pinch a little skin in which to insert the needle, which she did in a nice, steady way.

"Well done," I said, while Sarah's mother sighed in relief. (As did I!)

Sarah grinned from ear to ear and asked, "You do this all the time?"

"Every time."

She nodded understandingly.

For the majority of people, though, neither taking nor giving shots is anything they have very much experience with. And doing both at the same time? That's even stranger for most people. I try to keep this in mind whenever I'm about to administer myself a shot. I do multiple injection therapy, which is what most people living with type 1 diabetes do. Two long-acting insulin (basal rate) injections a day and a few short-acting (bolus) injections for meals. (The insulin pump, incidentally, is a form of multiple injection therapy.) And I try to take into account the cringe factor whenever other people happen to be around and I'll excuse myself and maybe give myself a shot in the restroom. But if I'm around friends who all know me, and we're somewhere doing something that I don't want to miss out on, I'll go ahead and give myself a shot on the spot. Of course, first I always ask if anybody minds. Nobody ever seems to. If they do, they're always free to look away at the crucial moment of injection. Do they? I never know because my attention is always focused on the injection!

The fact is, in addition to the day-to-day decisions you make as to when and where you take your shots, you should know how comfortable you are taking them in front of others. How well do you know the people you're about to give yourself an injection in front of? How will they react? Can you stay right there, or should you excuse yourself? The answers, of course, will depend on the situation and your assessment of the other people. As well, I might add, as to your own comfort level in being open with your condition.

Of course, with an insulin pump, you can be much more discreet than you can be with a syringe. You can pull the pump out and push a few buttons and, to the casual observer, it might look more like you're texting somebody than giving yourself insulin. Your only risk is appearing rude if you're in the middle of a conversation with someone. The pen can be more discreet than a syringe, too, since there's no vial and it looks more like a pen than a syringe.

One thing I've learned from experience: if you decide to give yourself your insulin (by pump, shot, or pen) in front of others, be prepared for questions. You'll get them. With my niece, I could turn her questions into a teaching moment. But sometimes I might just not be in the mood to answer questions and at those times I'll take my insulin in private.

The most frequently asked question I get? *Does it hurt?* "Sometimes," I reply. The second most common question seems to be, *how many shots do you take a day?* "Five to six." This is typically followed by the cringe factor and, many times, additional follow-up questions. People can be curious. So, if you're going to give yourself your insulin in front of others, you should be ready and willing to take the time to answer questions and educate others.

Some people are too nice to say anything, even if it bothers them to see someone inject him or herself with a needle. A few years back, my sister-in-law and her family came to live with us for several months while they were moving back to the United States from Holland, where they'd been living. I went about the house as usual, giving myself my injections whenever I needed them and thinking no more about it. Nobody seemed to mind. A year or so later, after my sister-in-law and her family had moved into their own home, they came over one evening for dinner. When it was just my sister-in-law and me alone together in the kitchen, I pulled out my syringe to give myself an injection, whereupon my sister-in-law promptly turned and walked out of the room. This, in mid-conversation.

"Hey, where are you going?" I managed to say, with the orange cap of the needle bobbing in my mouth, having just pulled it off with my teeth.

"I'm sorry, Gina," she said, "I'm uncomfortable watching you take your shot."

"But you saw me doing this for months!"

"I know." It turns out that while she was living with us, she'd been too polite to say anything.

What's interesting to me is that, having given myself injections since the age of seventeen, I apparently make it look easy, at least according to friends and family who have been witnesses. But of course, what they don't see is the work that goes on "behind the scenes." They don't see the process that takes place before the shot. The factors that I weigh. My carb ratio, my correction factor, my reaction time. What am I going to be eating? What have I just eaten? What kind of physical activity am I going to be engaged in? Or did I engage in? All the levers and pulleys. There's a lot that goes into that one single injection that someone might see me taking. The good thing for me is this: after all my years of experience, this process takes me no more than twenty or thirty seconds.

Now, once you know *when*, and you've taken into account your comfort level in giving your insulin around others to know *where*, then you have just one more decision to make, and it's another "where" question. Where on your body? This question is pertinent for a syringe, pen, or pump. In time, you'll discover your preferences. Your arm, your abdomen, your thigh, your buttocks. You should rotate the place of injection; using the same spot repeatedly can interfere with the absorption of your insulin. Even with a cannula, you'll want to move it around to allow previous insertion sites to heal. It's also important to realize that reaction times can vary depending on the spot of injection. In general, insulin is absorbed fastest in the abdomen, a little slower in the arms and legs, and slowest in the butt. As for me, I haven't noticed any measurable differences among the injection sites.

Over time, you'll find the areas that work best for you. For me, it's based mostly on convenience. In the summer, when I'm wearing shorts, perhaps, or short-sleeved tops, I'm more inclined to give myself an injection in the arms or legs. The abdomen is always convenient; you just lift your shirt. If I'm using the bathroom, it's often easiest to just take my injection in my butt.

Remember, the whole procedure is different for everybody. But as much as I preach personalization, there's one thing that's very black and white, and that's the fact that somewhere, somehow, you must take your insulin injections. There's no gray area where that's concerned.

At seventeen, I would not have believed that my taking of shots – multiple times a day – would be anything that could become so routine. In time, however, it did. Surprisingly, I learned that sticking yourself with a needle isn't as bad as it sounds. The dark side, as it turns out, isn't really all that dark after all. And the alternative (death!) makes it an easy choice.

7

Dining Well

Eat, Drink, & Enjoy Life

Let's talk about food. Of all the factors we've discussed thus far that you take into account as you begin to personalize the management of your chronic condition, perhaps nothing so directly affects your well-being as the food you eat.

For me, this means that by necessity I've become an expert label reader. If I'm going to be able to effectively anticipate how my body will react to what I'm planning on eating, then I need to know what's in it. And I mean *everything* that's in it. Fortunately, this is now getting easier. FDA requirements for labeling have become much more comprehensive. Not long ago, it wasn't uncommon to see "and additional spices" at the bottom of a list of ingredients on a food label. Now, those spices need to be identified. If you're living with celiac disease or are otherwise gluten intolerant, you'll appreciate this because some of those spices might well contain gluten.

My own general rule of thumb is to keep it simple. All things being equal, I'm always on the lookout for the food with the least amount of ingredients. That makes things easier. If I'm comparing bags of potato chips, I prefer to see nothing in the ingredients beyond "potatoes, salt, oil." Staying away from foods with lines and lines of listed ingredients cuts down on my chances of ingesting unwanted gluten or unwanted sugars. Extra ingredients collectively add up to just another variable to take into consideration with respect to how much insulin I'll need. It's all just additional noise that I'd rather do without.

More and more foods are labeled "Gluten Free" these days and of course that's extremely helpful to me. I look for GF foods. (Which I like to think means "Gina Friendly.") If I see two cans of soup and they both list the same exact ingredients, but one of them says "Gluten Free," I'll go with that one. The other might be gluten free as well, but I appreciate the fact that the first manufacturer took the time and effort to label their soup "Gluten Free." Even with a gluten-free label, though, I'm careful. My system doesn't tolerate gluten-free oats very well, for example. Many people living with celiac disease have no problem with GF oats, but I'm one of those people who does. But that's okay, because I know that and I can plan my meals accordingly.

And therein lies a key to food management that's just like all the management keys we've talked about so far: it comes down to personalization. Some foods might bother me but have no effect on you. And vice-versa. Rice is a challenge for me, for some unknown reason. It always makes my blood sugar rise no matter how I plan for it. No amount of accommodating by eating less of it, taking extra insulin, or a combination of the two seems to make a difference. I tried many times but finally just decided it's one of those quirky things I have to live with.

Dining Well

Or rather, I *don't* have to live with. Rice isn't that important to me, although I'll still eat it from time to time. When possible, I'll substitute. Maybe gluten-free pasta or fruit if available.

I call these foods "gotchas." Some might be obvious, but some may not be. In very general terms, you can assume foods sweeter in nature present a potential issue, although fruits less so than, say, cookies. Although both are simple carbs, fruits contain fiber, which helps slow down the digestion of carbs and reduces the likelihood of blood sugar spikes. You can accommodate with extra insulin, but added sugar tends to complicate matters and I prefer to keep things as uncomplicated as possible. Adding simple carbs like cookies into the mix makes the management of my diabetes just that much more challenging. As for more specific foods, you'll learn what disagrees with your system by experience and in time you'll have your own set of gotchas.

If you're having a blood sugar issue with any given food, your first course of action should be to check your carb ratio and portion size. Most of the time, just checking those two items will help you identify a potential problem. But, as with me and rice, there will still be gotcha foods regardless of carb ratio or portion size. It's why I take a couple of extra units of insulin for the Pancake Saturdays I mentioned earlier in the book. It happens that the carb count of my Pancake Saturday breakfast is the same as the carb count of my regular weekday breakfast. But I've learned that pancakes have more of an effect on my blood sugar. Hence the extra units. So, like everything we've discussed, it becomes a question of paying attention to what your body is telling you.

In fact, with time, avoiding gotchas becomes routine, even automatic. We have a natural tendency to gravitate towards the foods that agree with us, and away from the foods that are problematic. Case in point: out at dinner not long ago, a friend was asking about my blood sugar management and I mentioned the fact that there are certain foods that I try to avoid.

"Oh, is that why you haven't eaten all of your rice?" she asked. I looked down at my plate to discover a pile of rice that until that moment I hadn't consciously even seen. I'm sure on some level I knew the rice was there, but until this woman mentioned it, I had unwittingly been ignoring it.

As for portion size, learn to be a diligent label reader. Check out what the manufacturer considers a "serving size." You might be surprised at how small it is. A serving of breakfast cereal might not contain enough sugar, for instance, to be of concern, until you realize a serving is listed as half a cup and you normally eat three times that amount. Serving sizes vary, too, from manufacturer to manufacturer, making for some confusion.

Not to mention how easy it is, with certain foods, to pass right by the recommended serving without even noticing it. If you've ever sat down with a bag of potato chips, eating them unthinkingly in front of the TV, you know what I mean. In no time, you may have ingested four or five "servings." You should always be mindful of what you're eating and how much, making the appropriate insulin adjustments accordingly. This idea of mindfulness presents itself frequently at dinner parties. "Have some more!" a well-meaning host might say. But that doesn't necessarily mean you should. As with the Peanut Buster Parfait, sometimes a little caution is necessary with certain foods and a small taste is more than sufficient. Portion control is often the key.

In addition to the ingredients on a label, look at the "Nutrition Facts." The first item I look at is the carbohydrate content so that I can compensate appropriately with my insulin. Carbs come from starches, fiber, and sugars. I look at the total carb count, but it's also important to be aware that not all carbs are created equal. My body reacts to different carbohydrates differently. I'm more interested in how many carbs are coming from sugars than from fiber. Unlike simple sugars, fiber doesn't turn completely into glucose in the bloodstream. And complex carbohydrates – whole grains, vegetables – take longer to break down into glucose than simple sugars. There's no reason to avoid carbs. Carbs are energy. Just find the ones that work for you. Carbs in the form of potatoes work for me. I'm Irish, after all; potatoes are part of my DNA.

Of course, when you're dining out, the rules are a little different. You don't have labels to read, you just have a menu. So, you learn to estimate using experience and your best judgment. It's just another skill you develop over time for purposes of effective management. These days, many restaurants indicate which entrees are gluten free or low carb, so that makes ordering simpler than it used to be. For other concerns like carbs and sugar, you should use common sense. I have a rule of thumb I try to stick to at home and, for estimating purposes, it especially helps when I'm dining out. I mentally divide my plate in half and I make sure that one half contains nonstarchy vegetables (broccoli, asparagus, carrots, etc.). The second half gets mentally divided into two more parts, with one part (one-fourth of the plate) containing a carb (potato, pasta, rice, bread, fruit etc.), and the other part containing a protein (meat, cheese, or eggs, for instance). That's a good balance for me and the proportions seem to work well.

In some dining situations, you have less control over what's available to eat than in other situations. A small dinner party is an example. You and your significant other might be invited to have dinner with the boss and his or her spouse, for instance, where it's just the four of you, or maybe one other couple. Suppose there is exactly one choice for the main entree and maybe only a couple of choices for side dishes. And a sweet dessert that *everybody* is expected to partake in. At a large banquet,

The Nitty-Gritty of Managing Diabetes

these issues are no big deal. If I can't find a suitable option – either because of my celiac disease or because of a table full of gotchas that may play havoc with my blood sugar – I'll pull something out of my purse to eat. I *always* have something in my purse and for just such an emergency. And in a large room of people, nobody's going to take much notice of what I'm eating. Certainly, nobody's going to be offended if I pass on a certain food. In fact, I've experienced the opposite reaction – from people who have asked why I'm not eating the foods. It's both heartwarming and humorous to see several people dig into their backpacks, purses, and pockets in search of alternative food they might be carrying with them!

Sitting around someone's dining room table, however, can be more of a challenge. How to handle it? The best way is to not get yourself into such a predicament in the first place. There's absolutely nothing wrong with letting the host know beforehand, at the time when you accept the invitation, what dietary restrictions you might have. In fact, he or she will appreciate it. If it would be embarrassing for you to decline most of what's being offered for dinner, it would be just as embarrassing for the host. By knowing what you are comfortable eating, the host can accommodate your needs. Don't be afraid to speak up to avoid a potentially awkward moment. I'll even offer to help prepare or bring something, just to make the host's job even easier.

There's another frequent concern when eating out, and it hasn't anything to do with "eating." It's a rare banquet or dinner party or wedding or holiday meal that doesn't involve alcohol. "May I start you with a drink?" is often the first question out of a server's mouth. You can step into someone's home and have a glass of something thrust into your hand before you have your coat off. Sometimes going out with friends doesn't involve food at all: "Let's meet for a drink!"

Handling alcohol for a person living with diabetes or celiac disease is no different from handling food. It's just something else that needs to be *managed*. For my celiac disease, there are certain alcoholic beverages with gluten that I just simply choose not to drink – beers made with grains like malted barley and wheat, for example. Fortunately, today there are plenty of GF beers on the market brewed using millet, buckwheat, rice and/or corn. For my diabetes, I know that it's easier to manage if I stay away from sweet drinks. Daiquiris, sangria, mojitos – you can find a lot of sugar in these drinks, thus making them more challenging. My preference? Dry white wines. But that's me. You might enjoy something else.

Whatever you drink, it's important to realize how alcohol affects you. Will it make your blood sugar rise? Fall? You should drink responsibly. For me, I won't even indulge unless I've checked my blood sugar to confirm that it's in an acceptable range. If it's over 200 for instance, or below 70, I'll wait until it's somewhere around 100 to 150. I've learned from experience that, for me, if I drink alcohol when my blood sugar is around 200 or above, my blood sugar will keep rising. Conversely, if my blood sugar is below 70, it'll keep falling. And so, the 100 to 150 range is a good guideline for me. But your range might be different. Again, it's a case of personalization drawn from your own experience.

I'll also monitor my blood sugar after I have a drink to gauge the effects or to decide if I want a second drink. I'm reluctant to go much beyond that without a sufficient amount of time passing. Remember: you're in charge of managing your diabetes properly and you can't do that if you're impaired. You always need to be aware of your blood sugar level and able to make intelligent decisions about your insulin and food intake at all times. You wouldn't operate a car drunk and you shouldn't operate the management of your diabetes drunk, either.

Granted, this isn't always easy. There's always that well-meaning friend wanting to buy another round for everybody. Peer pressure isn't the issue for adults that it can be for young adults or teens, but sometimes it's still there. To avoid offending someone who sincerely just wants to offer up another drink, I'll often make sure I'm holding a full one. Maybe it's because I'm sipping my glass of wine very slowly, taking a good portion of the evening to drink it, or maybe it's because I'm holding a Diet Coke. Maybe it's even because I'm holding a dark-colored beer bottle that I've gone to the restroom to fill with water. In any event, I can claim honestly that, "I'm not ready for one yet, but thanks anyway!" Do whatever you're comfortable with doing.

It always helps to have a wingman along, too. (Or wingwoman.) Someone who knows you and understands your condition and limitations. Maybe you have a few too many. It happens. Doesn't hurt to have somebody along to remind you to check your blood sugar or eat something or even sit the next round out.

In the end, for me at least, it's more about the camaraderie than the drinking. "Are you having a good time?" a cousin of mine once asked me in a noisy Irish pub crowded with family.

"I'm having a great time!" I answered.

"What's that you're drinking?" she asked.

"A Diet Coke."

"You must be mad, Gina!"

It wasn't the first time I'd been accused of being crazy, and I could certainly understand my cousin's disbelief that I was sober yet having such an enjoyable time.

"Yep," I answered. "I can't help it. It's the company!" We laughed and my cousin understood: the drinking just wasn't that important to me.

A couple of summers ago I even participated in a "Twelve Pubs of Summer" pub crawl in Limerick, Ireland, on a vacation. It was a take-off on the "Twelve Days of Christmas," of course. We didn't get back to the hotel until 4:00 a.m. But all the while, I remained capable of managing my diabetes. First off, although a lot of people take the "twelve" literally, we figured four pubs were sufficient. Second, I drank slowly and ordered half-pints of cider when everybody else was ordering full pints of Guinness. Third, the length of the night afforded me a lot of time between drinks, time that I filled with water or Diet Coke. This allowed me to monitor my blood sugar regularly to make certain it was okay to imbibe some more or to eat something. And finally, I never lost sight of the fact that, for me, it was all about the people I was with and the atmosphere of the pubs. It was never about the pints of Guinness or about the half-pints of cider.

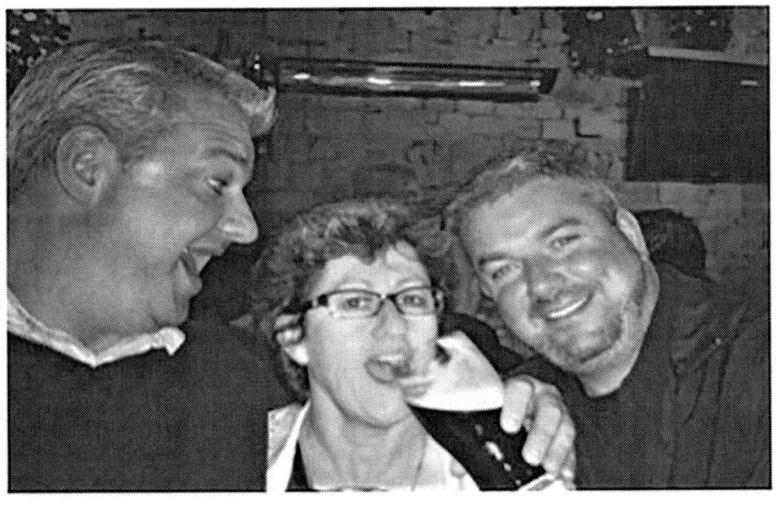

Me on a pub crawl in Limerick, Ireland with my cousins Shane and Darren. (No, I didn't drink the Guinness.)

By the same token, when dining out with friends, or family, or colleagues, it's never about the food. It's the social contact and the making of good times and good memories. I was reminded of this recently while giving a talk about living with diabetes and celiac disease. Someone in the audience asked what foods I miss the most. I thought back to high school where there was a diner that my friends and I would frequent late at night, after a movie or a party or a football game. Their specialty was a toasted corn muffin with melted butter. I haven't been able to find a substitute, especially a substitute for those mouth-watering muffins.

When I was sixteen, I went to work at a bakery. There, they had the best custard-filled donuts imaginable, with hard vanilla icing spread over them. I mean *the best*. A year later, I was diagnosed with diabetes. I still ate the donuts from time to time, but I've since moved. I think about them often, though, and I've never been able to find a decent substitute for them, either.

But in reminiscing about these foods from my past, I realized something. It wasn't the muffins or the donuts I really missed; it was the occasions when I ate them. The diner was a wonderful hangout where my friends and I would laugh and joke and talk about all the things that teenagers talk about. The bakery was another place of fond memories. It was an enjoyable job with fun coworkers. It's easy to make the mistake in both cases of thinking that the memories revolved around the food. And, yes, I certainly remember the taste of those muffins and donuts. But the truth is, the thing I miss the most is the camaraderie, the times I shared with my friends and colleagues.

Today, I'm making new memories with new friends and a lot of those memories happen to be set in restaurants or at dinner parties. Fancy restaurants, pubs, delis, cafés, breakfast eateries, banquet halls, or maybe somebody's home for the holidays. And though the occasion might revolve around a meal, it's never *about* the meal. It's about getting together with people whom you want to spend some quality time with. Once you remember that, having to be selective about what you eat becomes less important.

Above all else, don't become discouraged. I know what it's like to comb through a menu to find an entree you can (hopefully) eat while passing on all the delicious-sounding entrees you've chosen not to eat. For some people, it's overwhelming and they'd rather just stay home. Though understandable, this attitude is a pretty depressing way to go through life. Don't let caution become paralyzing to the point where you're afraid to leave the safe confines of your own kitchen. Take a chance. Go out and make some memories. Will you have missteps? Sure. Everybody does. But you learn from them and that just makes you even more knowledgeable about your condition(s). And acquiring more knowledge means gaining confidence, confidence that will enable you to put aside your anxieties and go out, eat, drink, and enjoy life!

8 Adventures Await You

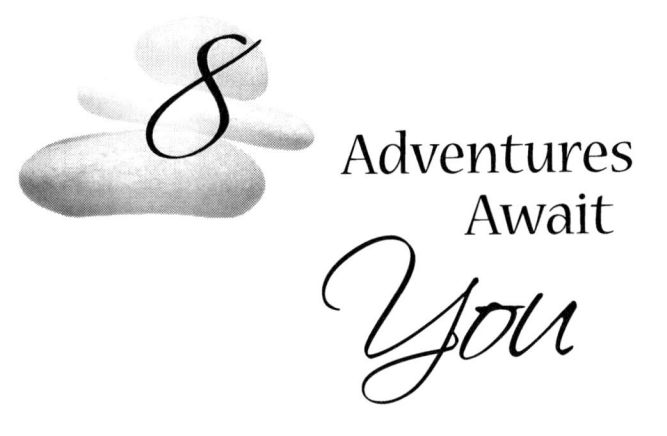

Being Confident Away from Home

Traveling can introduce a whole new set of levers and pulleys. Fortunately, I have some experience in this department. I've traveled around the United Kingdom, Germany, Ireland, Holland, China, Mexico, Canada, and throughout the U.S. For the most part, I try not to change the management of my diabetes very much at all. Sometimes that's hard. One potential snag is changing time zones. This can throw anybody off. My approach is to get myself on schedule with the new time zone as quickly as possible. On the way to my destination, I might take my long-acting insulin somewhere in between my regular time and the new (destination) time, splitting the difference. Then, when I arrive, I'll put myself on the new time right away. But I'll also test my blood sugar more frequently just to be sure.

On a long-distance flight, I'll typically take short-acting insulin more often (though in smaller doses). This allows for the fact that, over an extended period of time, sitting on a plane doing nothing very physical, your blood sugar will naturally rise.

Overall, I like to make sure I'm in what I call "what if" mode when I travel. What if something goes wrong? What if, for instance, my carry-on luggage gets lost, the luggage that I had my glucometer and syringes in? These are possibilities you need to prepare for. I always take two kits with me. That means an extra set of syringes, an extra glucometer and test strips, ketone strips, and extra insulin. It's a simple redundancy system that puts my mind at ease. If I'm traveling alone, I'll keep a kit in my purse and an exact duplicate in my carry-on. If Jim is traveling with me, I'll keep the extra kit in his carry-on.

If you're on the pump, think about what would happen if you somehow lost it along the way or it was stolen or malfunctions. Maybe you can get a replacement, but maybe not. Best case, it might take a day or so. What will you do in the meantime? You're probably not going to have another pump, so be prepared with syringes and both short-acting and long-acting insulin. Also, write down your current carb ratios, correction factor, and basal rates to assist you in being comfortable with returning to taking shots.

For celiac disease, eating out can present a problem when traveling because you'll most likely be going to restaurants that you're completely unfamiliar with. This unfamiliarity can become compounded if you're in a foreign country where the menu might be in a different language. Fortunately, from my own personal observations, the idea of "Gluten Free" (or "Celiac Friendly" as I've often seen it put in the UK) seems to have become fairly universal. You'll see it on menus everywhere, no matter the language.

Adventures Await You

Of course, you can always ask your server about a menu item, but that presupposes that you know their language or they know yours. Once, at a French restaurant in Quebec during a business visit with colleagues, I decided to ask the waitress about a particular entree but discovered that her understanding of English was limited. "Not so good," she responded when I asked about her English skills. I probably could have found something else to eat on the menu or pulled something from my bag, but the moment was saved by one of my colleagues who was fluent in both English and French. I explained to him my restrictions and to my surprise, he knew all about my condition. In fact, he touched his stomach and said, "Celiac disease?"

"Yes!" I said.

"I have a good friend who lives with celiac disease," he said. And then he proceeded to explain to the waitress exactly what the issue was. (And, for the record, the entree I ordered was *délicieux!*)

This is not the only time someone has come to my rescue at a foreign restaurant. On a couple of occasions, I've had English-speaking patrons, who happened to overhear my questions to the server, kindly jump in and translate for me. People are always willing to help no matter where in the world you find yourself.

But, just to be certain, there are websites – like this one: www.celiactravel.com/cards – where you can download cards that explain your requests to the server for you in whatever language is necessary.

Of course, it's always a good idea, no matter how far you're traveling, to carry some food or snacks with you. Don't always assume food will be readily available whenever you want or need it. What if you get stuck somewhere? What if your plane gets delayed or you end up lost traveling through another country?

And if there's one final piece of advice I could offer about traveling, no matter what your chronic condition might be, it would be this: do it! For me, I still have quite a few places on my bucket list, including Africa; Machu Picchu, Peru; Australia and New Zealand. There's a big world out there and you should never allow yourself to feel limited.

9 Leftovers

Miscellaneous Topics I'm Frequently Asked About

In my time as an author, advocate, and speaker, I've been asked many questions about living with diabetes and celiac disease. A lot of the questions, as you may imagine, have come from those who also live with one or both of those conditions (or other chronic conditions) and who are looking for practical advice. But many of the questions have also come from people who aren't living with any chronic condition at all but who are just naturally curious or wanting to support a family member or friend. I'm always pleasantly surprised at the level of interest from the latter group. But whatever their source, I'm always happy to help answer whatever questions come my way.

The Nitty-Gritty of Managing Diabetes

Since many of the questions don't necessarily require an entire chapter to answer, I thought it might be a better idea to group them together here. Think of these as leftovers, the questions we didn't really have an opportunity to address in the prior chapters.

I offer them to you here in no particular order:

> *If you were allowed to have just one condition – celiac disease or diabetes – which condition would you rather have?*

Um, could I pick none of the above? In truth, my answer to this question surprises a lot of people, especially people who are not all that familiar with the day to day management requirements of diabetes. Often, the perception is that you just watch what you eat (no sugar) and take your insulin. And so, when I say that, if given an option, I'd pick celiac disease (where your diet is even more limited) over diabetes, people are often thrown for a loop.

But my answer is not surprising to people who understand everything that's involved with the management of diabetes – all the levers and pulleys. Celiac disease has one lever: avoid gluten. Granted, that's not always easy to do. But the approach is at least simpler than diabetes. And the consequences aren't as severe, either. Gastrointestinal problems can be inconvenient, but not necessarily life-threatening, at least in the short term. If it isn't managed properly (if you keep eating gluten, in other words), celiac disease can lead to malnourishment, iron deficiency, osteoporosis, organ disorders, and even certain cancers. That's *if* it's not managed properly. On the other hand, with the threat of dangerously low blood sugar, diabetes can potentially be life-threatening in the very short term.

When I'm not eating, or planning to eat, I'm not thinking about my celiac disease at all. With my diabetes, on the other hand, I'm thinking about it all the time. I always need to be aware of my blood sugar level. It's a 24/7 proposition. Celiac disease is frustrating. Diabetes is challenging.

On the other hand, I must admit that my answer might be different if I was still a young girl. Children living with celiac disease can feel especially left out during childhood events like pizza parties and birthday parties with cake and other foods containing gluten. To a kid, celiac may be viewed as more confining than diabetes.

> *Would you have preferred that your diagnosis of diabetes had come later in life as opposed to earlier?*

On the surface, this seems like a no-brainer. Later, of course. But I was asked this question by a woman who was over forty and who had just recently been diagnosed. And I understood where her question came from. In a sense, she was almost envious of the fact that I was diagnosed at seventeen. This allowed me years to adapt, years she didn't have. I was able to learn all about the disease over an extended period of time. And when I was diagnosed, my lifelong behaviors hadn't been established yet. She had forty-plus years of eating and drinking habits she had to change. Lifetime routines were turned upside down. A lifestyle change was necessary.

All of this is true, I admit. On the other hand, as I explained to her, your management of diabetes changes over time because your body, indeed your life, changes over time. You never really get the chance to somehow become comfortable with any

The Nitty-Gritty of Managing Diabetes

given routine or set of behaviors. Whether you have forty years of experience behind you or four, you still never know exactly how your blood sugar is going to react on a daily basis. I'm still learning something new every day.

If there was any advantage at all to getting diagnosed younger, it might have been that the challenges forced me to become a stronger person in certain ways. Living with a chronic condition over time has made me a better problem-solver, more organized, more patient, and certainly more tolerant. But you know what? I would have loved to have had the opportunity to become all of those things on my own, without the help of diabetes, thank you very much.

How do you get past the resentment?

This is a very common question. And it's understandable. I'd venture that there's not a person who's ever lived with a chronic condition that, upon diagnosis, didn't scream, "Why me?" There's a lot of room for self-pity and I certainly spent my fair share of time wallowing in it.

But over time I've come to this conclusion: my chronic conditions are not hindrances. There's very little I can't do. Although I might not have seen it this way at the time, when I was diagnosed with them, my chronic conditions each represented a lifestyle change, nothing more. Sure, there's a lot more day-to-day maintenance involved in my life now than before my diagnoses. But it's nothing I can't handle.

Besides, everybody has something they are dealing with. Why me? Why *not* me? That's just life. My conditions might not be normal in the sense that most people don't have them. But that doesn't make *me* not normal. And what is normal, anyway? We're all different. We're all given different talents, different breaks, different challenges. We do the best we can, playing the cards we're dealt. To resent my conditions would be to resent the way that life works. Talk about banging your head against the wall! I have a lot of other pursuits in which I can direct my energy besides resentment and self-pity.

A quote from Mary Tyler Moore that I used in my first book *(There Is Something about Gina: Flourishing with Diabetes and Celiac Disease)* seems especially appropriate here: "Chronic disease, like a troublesome relative, is something you can learn to manage but never quite escape. And while each and every person who has type 1[diabetes] prays for a cure, and would give anything to stop thinking about it for just a year, a month, a week, a day even, the ironic truth is that only when you own it – accept it, embrace it, make it your own – do you start to be free of many of its emotional and physical burdens."

> *What happens if I'm with somebody who's living with diabetes and I witness them pass out or they seem as if they're about to pass out? What should I do?*

First, call 911. This can be a life-threatening situation. Second, treat the condition as if the person is suffering from *low* blood sugar, rather than high. If they're conscious, give them something with sugar immediately. A person living with diabetes can pass out from low or high blood sugar, but chances are good it's going to be from low. Why? Because high blood sugar is easier to see coming. There's more time to react. That means it's not as likely that the person losing consciousness is doing so because their blood sugar is high. Low blood sugar can take you by surprise. Sure, I can feel the effects if my blood sugar falls rapidly, say from 120 to 60 within an hour's time. But sometimes the fall can be so gradual that (if you're not monitoring yourself properly or just not paying attention) you won't notice until it's too late. For the record, in forty-plus years, I've never passed out from low blood sugar. But I have come close!

In fact, this idea of preventing low blood sugar is why I always keep some Life Savers with me – in my purse, in my pocket, in my coat, in my car, somewhere! A Life Saver is pretty discreet and easy to take out and pop in your mouth. I never go anywhere without them, whether it's on a long plane flight or a walk around the block. If ever I feel as though my blood sugar is falling, I'll reach for a Life Saver, which, if I'm really in trouble, may just live up to its name. For the same reason, some people carry glucose tabs with them. I prefer Life Savers but either way, it's all about being prepared.

What advice do you have for parents of children who are living with a chronic condition?

I get asked this quite often even though I'm always quick to point out that I am not a parent myself. Still, I feel I can at least offer a little advice that might be helpful. If nothing else, with the experience of having lived with my chronic conditions, maybe I can help provide the kid's point of view.

First, remember always that you are your child's biggest advocate. They need to know you support them and that no matter what, you'll always be there for them. That means educating yourself on your child's condition. You will want to become an expert. They'll be looking to you for guidance and answers. But you'll be learning together, collaborating, working as a team. The whole family is impacted by the condition of a child. And so, it's okay if you don't know everything. Together, you and your child can discover the answers.

You need to be patient with your child, too. They'll have setbacks and the setbacks will be frustrating for them. Don't add to the frustration. Kids seek approval and if they sense you're frustrated with a blood sugar reading, for example, it'll feel to them as though they've somehow failed. Do your best not to make them feel as though they're being graded. Remember how you felt when you were a kid? If your child comes to you with a problem only to get scolded or given a lecture, he or she will stop coming to you.

On the other hand, your child shouldn't be coddled, either. Much, of course, depends on the age of your child. Naturally, with a toddler, you're responsible for testing your child's blood sugar and injecting his or her insulin. But as your child gets older, their regular life responsibilities naturally increase and it shouldn't be any different with the management of their chronic condition. He or she will be an adult someday and will need to be prepared. The process of teaching responsibility and accountability is no different than how you'd progress any child into adulthood.

If you have other kids, make sure they understand and appreciate their sibling's condition. Keep them in the loop. Family support is crucial. Remember, however, that although it's natural to want to dote on the child who's living with a

The Nitty-Gritty of Managing Diabetes

chronic condition, be careful that your attention in that direction doesn't foster resentment in your other children. Yes, you may have to treat one child differently at times. Kids understand that, so long as, at the end of the day, everybody is treated *fairly*.

Above all else, I think it's important to remember that kids – all kids, no matter what – just want to be treated like any "normal" kid. A couple asked me one time about sending their teenage daughter to a summer camp for kids living with type 1 diabetes. These camps can be quite helpful. All the kids are there for the same reason and it's nice for the kids to be surrounded by others who understand their condition. Nobody has to explain themselves. Nobody asks what's on your arm (CGM) or why do you have tubing (insulin pump) or why are you pricking your finger (glucometer) or doesn't that hurt (shots)? This particular camp was a horse-riding camp. But there was another horse-riding camp, too, one that didn't specialize in kids living with diabetes.

"Do you think that it would be a good idea to send her to the diabetes camp?" these parents asked. "Because, for some reason, she seems pretty reluctant to go to that one."

"Well, how does she view herself?" I asked. "Does she consider herself a diabetic? Or does she consider herself as living with diabetes?"

"Oh," they replied, "she considers herself as living with diabetes. And she's managing it pretty well, though it could be better."

We talked a bit more and I gathered from the father that he was – no doubt with every good intention – micromanaging his daughter's condition. I could sense that she'd been feeling as though he was grading her. Seeking to avoid his disapproval, she'd even taken to timing her blood glucose tests to always get the best number. But overall, she was managing just fine. Although there were the typical aberrations, her hemoglobin A1C numbers were good.

I was sure the diabetes camp was valuable, but just not for this couple's daughter. "She's probably reluctant to go to the diabetes camp because she just doesn't want diabetes to be the focus," I offered. "And she just might not gain that much from such a camp at this point. She seems to be doing fine with managing her diabetes. Why not send her to the other camp?"

Later that summer I ran into the couple. Not only did the father adopt a more collaborative problem-solving approach with his daughter, they told me how much their daughter enjoyed the non-diabetes camp. Nobody there even talked about diabetes or seemed to care whether their daughter was living with diabetes or not. All anybody there cared about were the horses. And that was just fine with her. But much depends on your child's individual preference. Diabetes camps, non-diabetes camps—listen to your child and let him or her tell you what camp he or she thinks they will get the most out of.

Does your celiac disease affect your diabetes?

Unfortunately, yes. And that means it's yet another lever and pulley. Celiac disease presents its own problems, of course. But if you're not managing it properly, it can really create havoc with your blood sugar. If you're eating gluten, you won't be properly absorbing nutrients. And that means your blood sugar will be all over the place, which makes it extremely challenging to spot a trend or to make an informed adjustment.

For me, I discovered early on that if I eat gluten-free bread, I need to take an extra unit or two of insulin compared to bread with gluten ("gotcha"). Also, I tend to eat more fruit because of my celiac disease, as opposed to starches and carbs that may contain gluten. That affects my blood sugar, too. In the past couple years, however, I've gone back to eating more bread. Gluten-free bread is tasting better and better, and with a much better texture. There's even one brand that's so good that it's referred to around my house as a "gateway drug." Once I start eating it, lookout! I just *know* I'll have to adjust (take more insulin).

> *Do you believe there will be a cure for diabetes and/or celiac disease in your lifetime?*

In *my* lifetime? Unfortunately, I doubt it. But maybe future generations will benefit from a cure. What I think is more likely to happen is that some preventative measure, like a vaccine, will be discovered and the disease(s) will end up being slowly eradicated over time, much like polio. The vaccine won't help those already living with celiac disease or diabetes, but it will prevent others from getting them.

In the short term, I think we can always expect better treatments to come along. Technology is the key. Medical science is always progressing. For diabetes, keep in mind that insulin was only discovered in 1921, a relatively short time ago in the grand scheme of things. In my lifetime, I've seen a multitude of improvements in treatment options, especially in just the past few years. An example is the continuous glucose monitor that can interface with a pump. How long will it be before we have a totally closed-loop system where pumps do everything, sensing the blood-sugar level and automatically making the correct insulin adjustment? Probably not long.

In fact, coming out very soon is a hybrid system that can deliver a variable rate of basal insulin throughout the day that's based on your glucose reading from your CGM. This will enable better glucose control with reduced user input. You'll still be responsible for your bolus insulin, like at mealtimes for instance, and so it's not completely closed-loop, but we're obviously getting closer. These advances aren't cures, mind you. But the technology is advancing rapidly and each advance makes managing diabetes just a little easier.

For celiac disease (or at least gluten-intolerance), I've noticed a lot more awareness. Look at all the "GF" menus and labels these days. It's becoming more mainstream. And going forward, I expect that people will become even more aware. Eventually, I would expect some sort of treatment, perhaps some type of medication you can take that will allow your body to handle gluten with minimal side effects. There's always hope.

When it comes to managing diabetes, what are your thoughts about all the low-sugar and sugar-free alternatives in foods like ice cream and cookies?

We touched on this a little earlier in the book but I get asked about it so much that I think it deserves a little extra attention. On the surface, the sugar-free alternatives seem like a godsend to people who are living with diabetes. But a closer look at what goes into the alternatives can be a bit unsettling. Check out the label of a sugar-free dessert. You'll find a laundry list of chemical ingredients, most of which you can't even pronounce. I hold to the advice I mentioned earlier: keep it simple. If I'm buying ice cream, I don't want to see much more than "milk, cream, sugar." I'd rather make an insulin adjustment to accommodate the real stuff than to eat the stuff manufactured with substitutes. Plus, I'm willing to eat less of it, so long as it's real. Remember my Peanut Buster Parfait example? Sometimes just a couple spoonfuls are all you need.

I hear about "rebounding" a lot. What is this "rebounding"?

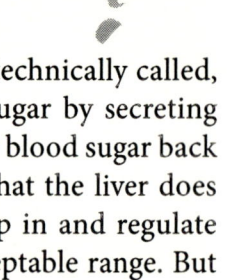

Rebounding, or the Somogyi effect, as it's technically called, is when the liver corrects for low blood sugar by secreting glycogen into the blood stream to raise your blood sugar back up again. So far so good. The problem is that the liver does this assuming the pancreas is going to step in and regulate the blood sugar level and keep it in an acceptable range. But of course, with someone living with type 1 diabetes, the pancreas does no such thing. The result? The blood sugar level just keeps rising.

For me, I've had times when my blood sugar was around 60 at dinner time. Too low. But after dinner, on towards bedtime, it was back up to 100 again. So everything seemed okay. But what I didn't see happening was that it was the rebounding effect that took the blood sugar to 100, and it wasn't going to stop there. By morning, it was all the way up to 260. Then I had to take extra insulin to get it back down. The danger, of course, is that if you're not careful, you'll find yourself suddenly on a roller-coaster you can't get off. Low, high, low, high, repeat.

Leftovers

If you're aware of the rebounding effect – and I am because for some reason I seem to be particularly susceptible to it – you can stop it before it gets too far along. For instance, in the above example, let's say I know my blood sugar has been considerably low (60). In this case, even though it might seem fine at bedtime (100), knowing about the rebounding effect, I'm going to take action anyway. I know my blood sugar is on the rise and so I might take an extra unit or two of insulin before I turn in for the night, thus (hopefully) preventing the high reading in the morning and keeping me off of the roller-coaster.

But of course, the best approach is to make sure your blood sugar level doesn't get too low to begin with. Then the liver minds its own business. And this underscores the importance of proper management, of being aware of where your blood sugar level is. And that, incidentally, makes this a situation in which the continuous glucose monitor can be quite helpful because you can spot the trends.

Okay, then what's the "dawn phenomenon"?

It's believed that blood sugar naturally rises in most people in the early morning hours. The dawn phenomenon refers to an abnormally high rise in some people living with diabetes. If this describes you on a regular basis, you might want to make a correction before bedtime, by adjusting your dosage, tweaking the time you take it, watching what you eat the night before, etc. The insulin pump is handy here. You can increase your basal rate for a few hours starting at, say, 4:00 a.m., when you're sleeping, to help combat the dawn phenomenon. Before you do anything, though, if you're experiencing the dawn phenomenon, you'll want to talk it over with your doctor.

The Nitty-Gritty of Managing Diabetes

> *What is the importance of the hemoglobin A1C test and why is my doctor so adamant that I have it?*

The hemoglobin A1C test is the gold standard for how your blood sugar is doing *over time*. It's a simple blood test that reflects your average blood sugar level over the past three months. It works because glucose binds to the hemoglobin in your red blood cells and red blood cells live for about three months. The test can measure, therefore, the amount of glucose built up over that time and provide an average. Averaging out the highs and lows allows you to make adjustments more accurately than a single reading here or there. And it reveals how you're trending in the long-term. Ideally, you should have a hemoglobin A1C test done every three months. You'll want to work closely with your doctor or medical team to best determine your target A1C. Remember, the numbers are important, but more important is the *trend*. Be patient and focus on going in the right direction.

> *I've heard that in certain cases, shortly after a diagnosis of type 1 diabetes, a person might go into remission. That sounds too good to be true. Is it?*

Yes, it is true, but the remission doesn't last. This period is referred to as the "honeymoon stage" and, although it didn't happen to me, I know people who experienced it. What happens is roughly this: in the early phase of the development of type 1 diabetes, a person's body still has some insulin-producing (beta) cells. The pancreas, in other words, still functions, even though the functioning is maybe only at a ten-percent level.

When the person starts taking insulin injections, demand on the pancreas is lessened. Thus "rested," the pancreas begins to produce insulin at a greater output. It's kind of a last hurrah. Sadly, the honeymoon stage doesn't last. Eventually, the process that destroyed most of the insulin-producing cells will destroy them all.

What's your opinion about consulting with a dietitian or nutritionist?

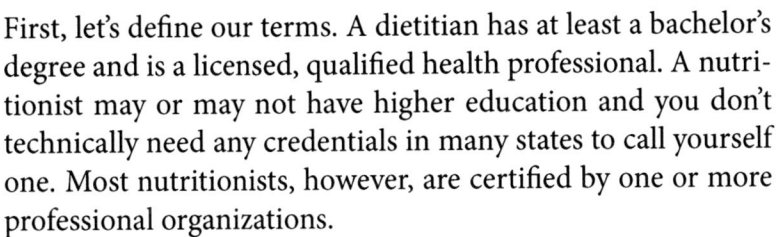

First, let's define our terms. A dietitian has at least a bachelor's degree and is a licensed, qualified health professional. A nutritionist may or may not have higher education and you don't technically need any credentials in many states to call yourself one. Most nutritionists, however, are certified by one or more professional organizations.

That said, either one can be helpful, depending on your individual needs. My first experience with a dietitian shortly after I was diagnosed with diabetes was not an especially good one. All she had to offer was a list of dietary do's and don'ts, a list I could easily have found by myself with five minutes of research at the library. And again, about five years ago, a dietitian just gave me a list, too. For me, I prefer expertise that is relevant for my particular situation and this requires a more consultative approach than handing me a list.

Whether it's a dietitian or nutritionist, I'll listen to anybody who has first listened *to me* and who therefore has a good handle on my needs. That way, I can get advice that has context behind it. This is not to say that lists are without any value. In fact, they can be extremely valuable. But, for me, I need to know how the lists relate to my specific set of circumstances. How can I actually make use of the information a list is imparting? That's the key.

How do you handle your diabetes when you're sick?

People living with diabetes should have a *sick day protocol* in place. An effective sick day protocol outlines what you can eat and drink, and how much. You need to remember that the management of your condition will change when you're ill. First, keep in mind that if you're vomiting and having trouble eating or drinking, your blood sugar will rise. Therefore, it's important to keep taking your insulin. And you should test your blood sugar more often. Your blood sugar will not be as predictable when you're ill. Don't assume – test! Every two or three hours, even through the night. It likely won't be at your usual level, but keep your blood sugar at least within reason.

Keep hydrated; drink plenty of fluids. Sports drinks, juices, and broths are good. Check your urine for ketones, too. Ketone is a chemical your body produces if there is a shortage of insulin. It indicates the body is beginning to break down fat to get energy. If there are too many ketones in your urine, call your doctor immediately. You can find ketone strips at your pharmacy. Always keep some on hand.

Keep emergency or after-hours phone numbers on hand, too, in case you need to reach your doctor at night or over a weekend or on a holiday. And never hesitate to have someone drive you to the emergency room if your condition begins to deteriorate or if you're just not bouncing back.

Ketones in the urine, blood sugar readings that continue to be too high, persistent diarrhea or vomiting, a fever that won't subside – these are all signals that medical help is necessary. If nothing else, you're most likely dehydrated, which is treatable in short order by a simple saline I.V. solution at your local hospital. Why wait?

More than anything, if you haven't discussed a sick day protocol with your medical team, make sure to do so. Don't wait until you're sick! Make sure you know what to do before you have to do it.

What's the role of family and friends?

Of course, I can only speak for myself, but my support group is extremely important to me. My husband, my friends, my family, my colleagues – anyone who understands my condition and who at one time or another has provided me with help or encouragement is a part of this group. Whether it's a reminder from Jim to check my blood sugar, a recommendation from colleagues as to a good place for lunch with lots of gluten-free menu choices, or just a family member/friend's sympathetic ear, it has always helped me enormously to surround myself with understanding people.

I consider my endocrinologist, and in fact my whole medical team, to be a part of this support group, too. I count on these people to advise me and to keep me informed on the latest medical developments relating to either or both of my conditions.

Interestingly, I have also found help from strangers or mere acquaintances. I mentioned earlier that I don't necessarily shy away from talking about my celiac disease or diabetes if someone who is genuinely curious asks me questions. And more than once, I've found myself pausing and looking at some element of one of my conditions in a new way because of a sincere question from someone who was on the outside looking in, someone with a more objective perspective. All in all, I've discovered that if you keep an open mind, you'll find help and support all around you.

10 Letting Nothing Get in *Your Way*

I hope, if you've gotten nothing else out of this book, you've learned the value of personalizing your approach to your chronic condition. But by so doing, you hopefully have also learned that personalizing means knowing yourself and knowing your condition. Only with these pieces of the puzzle can you put together an approach that is truly effective.

It all starts with the proper attitude. I know I said it earlier, but it's worth saying again: Life is meant to be enjoyed, experienced, and shared. Don't ever allow your chronic condition to get in your way. And staying away from the proverbial rabbit hole means, to a large degree, having confidence in your management abilities. So, learn all you can about your condition and – most importantly – about the ways of management that are right for you.

This means *knowing yourself* – and I encourage you to take some time to identify the type of personality you have. Remember Dr. Geil Browning's preferences for how people think? Are

The Nitty-Gritty of Managing Diabetes

you analytical, structural, social, or conceptual in your thinking? Or probably, like me, you're something of a combination. Having a good handle on how you process information will help you take the management path that's right for you.

Knowing yourself means knowing your body, and if you're living with type 1 diabetes, there are several factors that you need to become familiar with in so far as they affect you. Please review the many levers and pulleys we detailed earlier – major ones like your carb ratio, your correction factor, your reaction time to insulin, and your activity level. But also, learn about other factors that may affect you – your stress level, for example, or whether you have some illness you're battling. It takes patience, but in time, you'll learn from experience how the myriad of life's daily factors impacts you. Then you'll be better equipped to respond appropriately.

You'll want to review the tools that are available as well. For diabetes, there are many. Syringes, pens, pumps. Glucose monitors, continuous glucose monitors, CGMs that can interface with programmable pumps. Find the tools that work the best for you. For me, during the course of writing this book, I decided to go back on the pump. Mine interfaces with a CGM, the new game-changing technology we discussed earlier. I couldn't pass it up. And after a few weeks of wearing the pump, I've decided I'm okay with having it always tethered to me. In addition, I also now wear my CGM 24/7 rather than one week on, one week off.

But remember that whatever tools you decide to use, the management of your condition is still up to you. The tools might make it easier, but no tool has yet been invented that can replace a functioning pancreas. And until one is, the management of your diabetes ultimately rests with you.

Food is a key factor, of course. Know the food you put into your body. Learn to be a careful, patient label reader. At restaurants, don't be afraid to ask for clarification on menu items you're unsure about. Know your gotchas. Understand how your body processes alcohol. Most of all, don't let your condition hold you back from enjoying yourself!

And therein lies perhaps the most important lesson I'd like to impart as I close this book. A chronic condition (or, as in my case, chronic condition*s*) need not stop you from living your life the way you want to live it. Do you have to live with a few limitations? Well, yes. Do you have to plan a little more? Sure. But in the larger picture, that's just life. We all have circumstances or situations, chronic or otherwise, that we must deal with every day. The key is to find solutions, or at least workarounds, so that those circumstances or situations won't stop us. Your workarounds might be different than mine, and that's okay, and to be expected. When we're both diligent, we'll both end up in the same place – enjoying, experiencing, and sharing life. And letting nothing get in our way.

I said this to end my first book and it warrants being said again: Life awaits you, with all of its wonders. All you have to do is decide that, just for today, nothing's going to stop you.

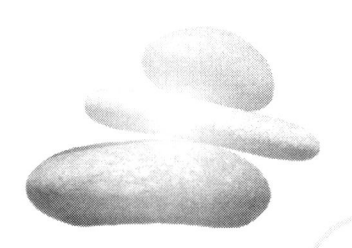

Epilogue

At the age of seventeen, I was diagnosed with diabetes. At the age of thirty-two, I was diagnosed with celiac disease. At the age of fifty-seven, I was diagnosed with heart disease.

It's difficult not to wonder what's next! But if I've learned anything from the first two diagnoses, it's that worrying too much about the future is time-wasting. Having to overcome the hurdles that both diabetes and celiac disease present me with has ultimately led me not to a place of resentment, but one of gratitude. There's no way around it, really. If you're going to move forward, you have to decide to be thankful for all that you have that is good.

With my heart issue, this attitude was only confirmed. Alas, I must confess that such was not the case at first. The physical aspect of my recovery was time-consuming, but steady. The emotional aspect was something else entirely. I was, to put it mildly, completely unprepared to deal with what happened to me. I was even less prepared to deal with the thoughts of what

The Nitty-Gritty of Managing Diabetes

could have happened to me. Without my diagnosis and treatment, I would have been mere weeks away from a heart attack. Maybe a fatal one.

What I initially felt was a kind of vulnerability. I was mortal. I found myself with a strange lack of confidence. What if something else happens, I wondered? Would I even be able to deal with it? I was anything but certain.

I was afraid.

But time, they say, heals all wounds and in my case, it also removed a lot of the doubt. Little by little, as I gained my physical strength back, a process that took more than a year, I also gained back my confidence. At first, I was tentative. When I finally got back on the basketball court, I found myself playing cautiously, careful not to exert myself. A pass slightly out of reach? I'd let it go. The chance of a rebound if I got aggressive? I'd defer to a teammate.

Weeks and months went by. I tried to push myself as best I could. Then one day, in the middle of a game, a pass was thrown way over my head and out of bounds. I instinctively turned and ran after the ball, grabbing it and running back to the court to put it in play. Suddenly it hit me what I had just done.

"Did you guys just see that?!" I said. "Did you see the way I just hustled after the ball?!"

It was a crowning moment. I knew in an instant that I was back. In one spontaneous, unconscious act, I had proven that I was okay again. Really okay. And at that moment I was struck with a tremendous feeling of gratitude that stays with me still.

I don't want to lose that feeling. I've determined that I'm not going to waste any time feeling anything less than appreciative for every day. I've retired from my day job since I started this book, something I was considering anyway. But the events of the past couple of years moved the timetable up a bit. Jim and I have a lot we want to do now, including a list of places we want to travel to. But even on days with nothing planned, we take advantage of the time, going on hikes around the neighborhood that just a year or so ago I could barely walk around. Smelling the proverbial roses is what we're doing, although in our case, it's the lilac bushes in our yard.

What I learned through my heart condition was something I'd learned to a lesser degree with my diabetes and celiac disease: life is meant to be lived and enjoyed and there's really no time to let anything stand in the way of that. I knew that all along, of course, and I suspect we all do on some level. But for me, it took something as life-altering as a potentially fatal heart attack to really drive it home. I hope it doesn't take something quite as dramatic for you!

Now that you're done reading, put the book down, take a long walk, and smell some roses or lilacs or just the dynamic air of possibilities offered by another day of living. Be present. Most of all, be grateful.

~ *Gina*